T0205239

METHODS IN MOLECULAR BIOLOGY

Series Editor
John M. Walker
School of Life and Medical Sciences
University of Hertfordshire
Hatfield, Hertfordshire, AL10 9AB, UK

For further volumes:
http://www.springer.com/series/7651

Intravital Imaging of Dynamic Bone and Immune Systems

Methods and Protocols

Edited by

Masaru Ishii

Department of Immunology and Cell Biology, Graduate School of Medicine,
Osaka University, Osaka, Osaka, Japan

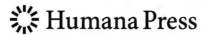 Humana Press

Editor
Masaru Ishii
Department of Immunology and Cell Biology
Graduate School of Medicine, Osaka University
Osaka, Osaka, Japan

ISSN 1064-3745   ISSN 1940-6029   (electronic)
Methods in Molecular Biology
ISBN 978-1-4939-8544-9   ISBN 978-1-4939-7762-8   (eBook)
https://doi.org/10.1007/978-1-4939-7762-8

Printed on acid-free paper

This Humana Press imprint is published by Springer Nature
The registered company is Springer Science+Business Media, LLC
The registered company address is: 233 Spring Street, New York, NY 10013, U.S.A.

Preface

During the last decade, advanced intravital imaging technology by using multiphoton excitation fluorescent microscopy has revolutionized the field of biological sciences. Based on these techniques, we are now able to visualize in situ behavior of a diversity of living cells "intravitally" within intact tissues and organs. This research trend would be quite meritorious especially for analyzing bone and immune systems, where various kinds of cell types are moving around and their spatiotemporal control is pivotal for proper functions in vivo. For example, bone is a mysterious organ where various kinds of hematopoietic and immune cells are produced and functioning although poorly analyzed by conventional methodology such as histological analyses with decalcified bones. Intravital imaging of bones has identified the behavior of bone cells such as osteoclasts, specialized macrophages contributing to bone destruction, revealing novel mechanisms controlling their migration and function in situ. Furthermore, visualization of the dynamic movement of various cell types in lymph nodes, skin, kidney, nervous systems, and cancer tissues has identified crucial mechanisms and factors triggering their migration and infiltration in these areas.

Despite the increased importance of the methods in biological sciences and the availability of expensive imaging modalities such as multiphoton microscopy in many research institutes, one of the big hurdles preventing popularization of this research trend has so far been the complicated experimental protocol. Researchers need the procedures to be elaborated for themselves in their respective laboratories.

In this book, leading researchers who are actually doing imaging studies in the field of bone and immune systems contributed the chapters where they described respective actual cutting-edge protocols, including some "secret recipes." These detailed methods would surely be useful for general readers in order to establish and perform these experiments on their own.

I express my sincere gratitude to all the authors for their willingness to share their secrets and to Prof. John Walker at Humana Press for giving me the opportunity to publish this book for the series. Both he and the authors have been patient during the editing of this volume.

Osaka, Japan   *Masaru Ishii*

Contents

Contributors

TSUYOSHI AKAGI • *KAN Research Institute Inc., Kobe, Hyogo, Japan*

CLEMENS ALT • *Center for Systems Biology and Wellman Center for Photomedicine, Massachusetts General Hospital and Harvard Medical School, Boston, MA, USA*

MARC BAJÉNOFF • *Aix-Marseille University, Centre National de la Recherche Scientifique (CNRS), Institut National de la Santé et de la Recherche Médicale (INSERM), Centre d'Immunologie de Marseille-Luminy (CIML), Marseille, France*

PIERRE C. DAGHER • *Division of Nephrology, Department of Medicine, Indiana University, Indianapolis, IN, USA*

GYOHEI EGAWA • *Department of Dermatology, Kyoto University Graduate School of Medicine, Kyoto, Japan*

BRIAIRA GEIGER • *Department of Chemistry, Richard Stockton College of New Jersey, Galloway, NJ, USA*

REBECCA GENTEK • *Aix-Marseille University, Centre National de la Recherche Scientifique (CNRS), Institut National de la Santé et de la Recherche Médicale (INSERM), Centre d'Immunologie de Marseille-Luminy (CIML), Marseille, France*

CLÉMENT GHIGO • *Aix-Marseille University, Centre National de la Recherche Scientifique (CNRS), Institut National de la Santé et de la Recherche Médicale (INSERM), Centre d'Immunologie de Marseille-Luminy (CIML), Marseille, France*

CHI CHING GOH • *Singapore Immunology Network (SIgN), A*STAR (Agency for Science, Technology and Research), Singapore, Singapore; Department of Microbiology, Immunology Programme, Yong Loo Lin School of Medicine, National University of Singapore, Singapore, Singapore*

TAKASHI HATO • *Department of Medicine, Indiana University, Indianapolis, IN, USA*

TETSUYA HONDA • *Department of Dermatology, Kyoto University Graduate School of Medicine, Kyoto, Japan*

MATTEO IANNACONE • *Division of Immunology, Transplantation and Infectious Diseases, IRCCS San Raffaele Scientific Institute, Milan, Italy; Vita-Salute San Raffaele University, Milan, Italy; Experimental Imaging Center, IRCCS San Raffaele Scientific Institute, Milan, Italy*

WATARU IKEDA • *KAN Research Institute Inc., Kobe, Hyogo, Japan*

MASARU ISHII • *Department of Immunology and Cell Biology, Graduate School of Medicine, Osaka University, Osaka, Japan*

YOOKYUNG JUNG • *Center for Systems Biology and Wellman Center for Photomedicine, Massachusetts General Hospital and Harvard Medical School, Boston, MA, USA; Center for Molecular Spectroscopy and Dynamics, Institute for Basic Science (IBS), Seoul, Republic of Korea*

KENJI KABASHIMA • *Department of Dermatology, Kyoto University Graduate School of Medicine, Kyoto, Japan*

TOMOYA KATAKAI • *Department of Immunology, Graduate School of Medical and Dental Sciences, Niigata University, Niigata, Japan*

NAOTO KAWAKAMI • *Institute of Clinical Neuroimmunology, University Hospital and Biomedical Center, Ludwig-Maximilians University Munich, Munich, Germany; Max-Planck Institute of Neurobiology, Martinsried, Germany*

JUNICHI KIKUTA • *Department of Immunology and Cell Biology, Graduate School of Medicine, Osaka University, Osaka, Japan*

MIRELA KUKA • *Division of Immunology, Transplantation and Infectious Diseases, IRCCS San Raffaele Scientific Institute, Milan, Italy; Vita-Salute San Raffaele University, Milan, Italy*

JACKSON LIANGYAO LI • *Singapore Immunology Network (SIgN), A*STAR (Agency for Science, Technology and Research), Singapore, Singapore; School of Biological Sciences, Nanyang Technological University, Singapore, Singapore; CNIC (Fundación Centro Nacional de Investigaciones Cardiovasculares), Madrid, Spain*

CHARLES P. LIN • *Center for Systems Biology and Wellman Center for Photomedicine, Massachusetts General Hospital and Harvard Medical School, Boston, MA, USA*

SAYAKA MATSUMOTO • *Department of Immunology and Cell Biology, Graduate School of Medicine, Osaka University, Osaka, Japan*

RYOHEI MATSUURA • *Department of Cardiovascular Surgery, Osaka University, Graduate School of Medicine, Osaka, Japan*

SHIGERU MIYAGAWA • *Department of Cardiovascular Surgery, Osaka University Graduate School of Medicine, Osaka, Japan*

MASAYUKI MIYASAKA • *MediCity Research Laboratory, University of Turku, Turku, Finland; Interdisciplinary Program for Biomedical Sciences, Institute of Academic Initiatives, Osaka University, Suita, Osaka, Japan*

LAI GUAN NG • *Singapore Immunology Network (SIgN), A*STAR (Agency for Science, Technology and Research), Singapore, Singapore; School of Biological Sciences, Nanyang Technological University, Singapore, Singapore; Department of Microbiology, Immunology Programme, Yong Loo Lin School of Medicine, National University of Singapore, Singapore, Singapore*

SATOSHI NISHIMURA • *Research Division of Cell and Molecular Medicine, Center for Molecular Medicine, Jichi Medical University, Tochigi, Japan*

ANTHONY P. RAPHAEL • *Center for Systems Biology and Wellman Center for Photomedicine, Massachusetts General Hospital and Harvard Medical School, Boston, MA, USA; Dermatology Research Centre, Translational Research Institute, School of Medicine, The University of Queensland, St Lucia, QLD, Australia*

ANDREA REBOLDI • *Department of Pathology, University of Massachusetts Medical School, Worcester, MA, USA*

JUDITH R. RUNNELS • *Center for Systems Biology and Wellman Center for Photomedicine, Massachusetts General Hospital and Harvard Medical School, Boston, MA, USA*

ASUKA SAKATA • *Research Division of Cell and Molecular Medicine, Center for Molecular Medicine, Jichi Medical University, Tochigi, Japan*

STEFANO SAMMICHELI • *Division of Immunology, Transplantation and Infectious Diseases, IRCCS San Raffaele Scientific Institute, Milan, Italy; Vita-Salute San Raffaele University, Milan, Italy*

KEN SASAI • *KAN Research Institute Inc., Kobe, Hyogo, Japan*

YOSHIKI SAWA • *Department of Cardiovascular Surgery, Osaka University Graduate School of Medicine, Osaka, Japan*

JOEL A. SPENCER • *Center for Systems Biology and Wellman Center for Photomedicine, Center for Regenerative Medicine, Massachusetts General Hospital and Harvard Medical School, Boston, MA, USA; School of Engineering, University of California Merced, Merced, CA, USA*

AKIRA TAKEDA • *MediCity Research Laboratory, University of Turku, Turku, Finland*

MICHIO TOMURA • *Laboratory of Immunology, Faculty of Pharmacy, Osaka Ohtani University, Osaka, Japan*

EIJI UMEMOTO • *Laboratory of Immune Regulation, Department of Microbiology and Immunology, Osaka University Graduate School of Medicine, Suita, Osaka, Japan*

SETH WINFREE • *Department of Medicine, Indiana University, Indianapolis, IN, USA*

JUWELL W. WU • *Center for Systems Biology and Wellman Center for Photomedicine, Massachusetts General Hospital and Harvard Medical School, Boston, MA, USA*

Chapter 1

Bone Imaging: Osteoclast and Osteoblast Dynamics

Junichi Kikuta and Masaru Ishii

Abstract

Bone is continually remodeled by bone-resorbing osteoclasts and bone-forming osteoblasts. Although it has long been believed that bone homeostasis is tightly regulated by communication between osteoclasts and osteoblasts, the fundamental process and dynamics have remained elusive. To resolve this, we established an intravital bone imaging system using multiphoton microscopy to visualize mature osteoclasts and osteoblasts in living bone.

We herein describe the methodology for visualizing the in vivo behavior of bone-resorbing osteoclasts and bone-forming osteoblasts in living bone tissues using intravital multiphoton microscopy. This approach facilitates investigation of cellular dynamics in the pathogenesis of bone-destructive disorders, such as osteoporosis and rheumatoid arthritis in vivo, and would thus be useful for evaluating the efficacy of novel anti-bone-resorptive drugs.

Key words Intravital imaging, Multiphoton microscopy, Osteoclast, Osteoblast, pH-sensing probe

1 Introduction

Bone is a dynamic tissue that undergoes continuous remodeling by bone-resorbing osteoclasts and bone-forming osteoblasts [1]. Tight control of bone remodeling is critical for maintaining bone homeostasis in response to structural and metabolic demands. Bone remodeling is strictly controlled through a complex communication network between osteoblast- and osteoclast-lineage cells [2]. Therefore, it is essential to understand the spatial–temporal relationship and interactions between osteoblasts and osteoclasts in vivo. In particular, it remains controversial whether these cell types physically interact with each other.

Bone is the hardest tissue in the body; for this reason, it is technically difficult to visualize cellular interactions in the bone marrow cavities of living animals. The morphology and structure of bone tissues can be analyzed using various conventional methods, including micro-computed tomography, histomorphological analyses, and flow cytometry. These methods yield information on cell shape and gene expression patterns, but not on dynamic cell movements in living bone marrow. The recent introduction of fluorescence microscopy has enabled imaging of the cellular dynamics of organs and tissues in vivo [3, 4]. Therefore, we established an advanced imaging system to visualize living bone tissues using intravital multiphoton microscopy [5–8]. For visualization of deep bone tissue, we selected the parietal bone of mice, which is ~80–120 μm thick (within the range of infrared lasers), as the observation site. In this region, living bone marrow can be accessed with minimal invasion.

To visualize mature osteoclasts (mOCs), we generated transgenic reporter mice expressing tdTomato, a red fluorescent protein, in the cytosol of mOCs (TRAP-tdTomato mice) [8]. To visualize mature osteoblasts (mOBs), we also generated fluorescent reporter mice expressing enhanced cyan fluorescent protein (ECFP) in the cytosol of mOBs (Col2.3-ECFP mice). To visualize communication between mOCs and mOBs, we crossed TRAP-tdTomato mice with Col2.3-ECFP mice to generate TRAP-tdTomato/Col2.3-ECFP double fluorescently labeled mice. Using intravital multiphoton microscopy of calvaria bone tissues of TRAP-tdTomato/Col2.3-ECFP mice, we successfully visualized the in vivo behavior of living mOCs and mOBs on the bone surface; the imaging results suggested direct interactions between mOCs and mOBs in vivo. In wide views of skull bones under normal conditions, mOCs and mOBs appeared to be distributed separately, although some direct, albeit spatiotemporally limited, mOC–mOB interactions were evident. Analysis of time-lapse images showed that mOCs and mOBs exhibited distinct spatial distributions. However, several mOCs in contact with mOBs displayed dendritic shapes and projected synapse-like structures toward mOBs. Additionally, these interactions between mOCs and mOBs changed dynamically according to bone homeostatic conditions.

We recently developed pH-sensing chemical fluorescent probes to detect localized acidification by bone-resorbing osteoclasts on the bone surface in vivo [9, 10]. These probes are based on the boron-dipyrromethene (BODIPY) dye and a bisphosphonate group. BODIPY dyes have a large number of applications because of their environmental stability, large molar absorption coefficients, and high fluorescence quantum yields [11]. The bisphosphonate group replaces phosphate ions in hydroxyapatite, the main component of bone tissue, and forms a tight bond with the bone matrix. Therefore, the bisphosphonate group facilitates delivery and fixation of the probe on bone in living animals [12]. Our recently developed pH-probes enabled visualization of bone resorption by osteoclasts, which led to identification of two distinct functional states of differentiated osteoclasts: bone-resorptive [R] and non-resorptive [N].

In this chapter, we describe a methodology for visualizing the in vivo behavior of osteoclasts and osteoblasts simultaneously in living bone tissue. In addition, we describe imaging of osteoclast function using a pH-sensing fluorescent chemical probe.

2   Materials

2.1   Multiphoton Microscopy

2.1.1   Standard Imaging

1. Upright multiphoton microscope (A1R-MP; Nikon) (*see* **Note 1**).

2. Water-immersion objective, 25× (APO: numerical aperture [NA], 1.1; working distance [WD], 2.0 mm; Nikon) (*see* **Note 2**).

3. Femtosecond-pulsed infrared laser (Chameleon Vision II Ti: sapphire laser; coherent) (*see* **Note 3**).

4. External non-descanned detector (NDD) with four channels (Nikon).

5. Dichroic and filter set: Three dichroic mirrors (458, 506, and 561 nm), and four band-pass filters (417/60 nm for the second harmonic generation (SHG) signal, 480/40 nm for ECFP, 534/30 nm for autofluorescence, and 612/69 nm for tdTomato) (Nikon) (*see* **Note 4**).

6. NIS Elements integrated software (Nikon).

2.1.2   Spectral Imaging (*See* **Note 5**)

1. Upright multiphoton microscope (LSM 780 NLO; Carl Zeiss).

2. Water-immersion objective, 20× (W Plan-Apochromat: NA, 1.0; WD, 2.4 mm; Carl Zeiss).

3. Femtosecond-pulsed infrared laser (Chameleon Vision II Ti: sapphire laser; coherent).

4. Internal 32-channel GaAsP spectral detectors (Carl Zeiss).

5. ZEN software (Carl Zeiss).

2.2   Mice and Anesthesia

1. TRAP-tdTomato [8] and Col2.3-ECFP mice.

2. Isoflurane (Escain).

3. Vaporizer (inhalation device).

4. O_2 bomb.

5. Anesthesia box and mask.

2.3   Intravital Imaging

1. Custom-made stereotactic stage (Fig. 1) (*see* **Note 6**).

2. Head holder with a hexagonal window (*see* **Note 7**).

3. Shaver and hair-removal lotion.

4. Iris scissors and tweezers for mouse surgery.

5. *N*-Butyl cyanoacrylate glue.

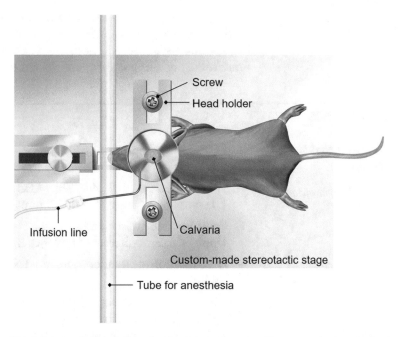

Fig. 1 Schematic illustration of calvaria bone imaging. The mouse is anesthetized with isoflurane, the frontoparietal region of the skull bone is surgically exposed, and its head is immobilized using the custom-made stereotactic holder. The head holder is kept fully loaded with PBS by an infusion syringe pump

6. Ethyl-cyanoacrylate glue.

7. Infusion line.

8. Infusion syringe pump.

9. Phosphate-buffered saline (PBS) buffer, pH 7.4.

10. Electrocardiogram monitoring device.

11. Environmental dark box in which an anesthetized mouse is warmed to 37 °C by an air heater.

2.4 Preparation of the pH-Sensing Probe

1. pH-sensing chemical fluorescent probe (Fig. 2) [10].

2. PBS immersion buffer, pH 7.4.

3. One 26-gauge needle.

2.5 Staining of Blood Vessels

1. Angiographic agent: Qtracker 655.

2. One 29-gauge insulin syringes for intravenous injection.

2.6 Image Processing and Analysis

1. Image processing and analysis software: Imaris (Bitplane), NIS Elements (Nikon), and ZEN (Carl Zeiss).

2. After Effects software (Adobe).

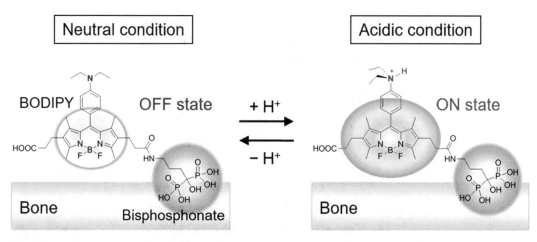

Fig. 2 Chemical structure of the pH-sensing fluorescent chemical probe. The pH-sensing probe is based on the boron-dipyrromethene (BODIPY) dye for visualization in low-pH environments in bone created by active osteoclasts; the bisphosphonate group facilitates delivery of the probe to bone tissue. Fluorescence of the probe can be detectable under acidic condition

3   Methods

3.1   Administration of the pH-Sensing Probe

1. Dissolve 5 mg/kg of pH-sensing chemical probe (pHocas-3) in PBS.
2. All procedures in mice are performed under anesthesia.
3. Inject the pH-probe subcutaneously into mice daily beginning 3 days prior to imaging.
4. Perform intravital bone imaging experiments (*see* Subheading 3.2).

3.2   Intravital Multiphoton Imaging of Calvaria Bone

1. Start up the multiphoton microscope and turn on the heater in the environmental dark box (*see* **Note 8**).
2. All surgical procedures are performed under isoflurane inhalation anesthesia.
3. Shave the hair and apply hair-removal lotion to the top of the head of the mouse (*see* **Note 9**).
4. Disinfect the skin of the head using 70% ethanol.
5. Cut the skin minimally using iris scissors and then expose the frontoparietal region of the skull.
6. Resect marginal muscles and the periosteum.
7. Apply *n*-butyl cyanoacrylate glue to the back of the head holder.
8. Apply ethyl-cyanoacrylate glue to the marginal area of the exposed bone, but not to the skull bone within the hexagonal window.

9. Place the head holder on the skull bone using the skull bone suture as an anatomical landmark.

10. Wait a few minutes to allow the glue to firmly secure the skull bone to the head holder (*see* **Note 10**).

11. Fix the head holder to the custom-made stereotactic stage using two screws, and immobilize the mouse as tightly as possible to avoid drift secondary to respiration and pulsation (Fig. 1) (*see* **Note 11**).

12. Set the infusion line in the groove of the head holder, and fill the hexagonal window with PBS (*see* **Note 12**).

13. Place the mouse in the environmental dark box.

14. If necessary, intravenously inject Qtracker 655 dissolved in PBS.

15. Focus on the bone marrow cavity at an appropriate depth and look through the ocular lenses using a mercury lamp as the light source.

16. Change the light source from the mercury lamp to the Ti: sapphire laser.

17. Set the excitation wavelength, zoom ratio, z-positions, interval time, and duration time using the microscope software (*see* **Note 13**).

18. Observe the bone tissue by multiphoton excitation microscopy.

19. Monitor the heart rate of the mouse using an electrocardiogram throughout imaging (*see* **Note 14**).

3.3 Image Processing and Analysis

1. Obtain the SHG, autofluorescence, pHocas-3, ECFP, and tdTomato fluorescence spectra from the raw images using ZEN software by manually selecting appropriate pixels.

3.3.1 Spectral Unmixing for Images Acquired by 32-Channel GaAsP Spectral Detectors

2. Utilize these spectral libraries for spectral unmixing algorithms.

3. Discriminate each fluorescence signal, exclude autofluorescence, and create unmixed images (Fig. 3).

3.3.2 Analysis of Intravital Multiphoton Images

1. Correct images for XY drift using NIS Elements or Imaris software.

2. Analyze images by measuring the frequency and duration of cell-to-cell contact using Imaris software (Fig. 4).

3. Create the movie using After Effects software.

4   Notes

1. There are two types of microscope: upright and inverted. Bone marrow can be observed using an inverted microscope. Multiphoton microscopes are also available from other manufacturers (e.g., Leica Microsystems and Olympus).

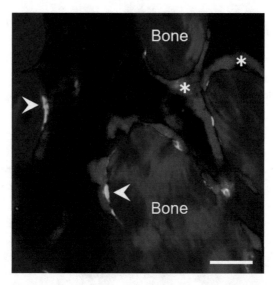

Fig. 3 Visualization of the bone-resorptive function of mature osteoclasts using a pH-sensing fluorescent probe. Representative images of the calvaria of TRAP-tdTomato mice treated with a pH-probe, showing sites of local bone resorption. Red, mature osteoclasts expressing TRAP-tdTomato; green, fluorescence signals from areas of high H$^+$ concentration; blue, bone tissue. Arrowheads and asterisks represent bone-resorptive and non-resorptive osteoclasts, respectively. Scale bar, 40 μm

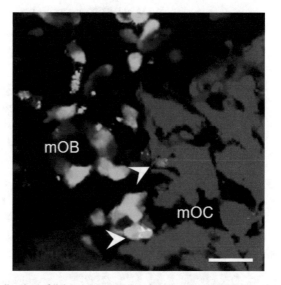

Fig. 4 Visualization of living mature osteoclasts and osteoblasts on bone surface by intravital multiphoton microscopy. Representative image of the calvaria of TRAP-tdTomato/Col2.3-enhanced cyan fluorescent protein (ECFP) mice under control conditions. Red, mature osteoclasts (mOCs) expressing TRAP-tdTomato; cyan, mature osteoblasts (mOBs) expressing Col2.3-ECFP. Arrowheads represent mOB–mOC interactions. Scale bar, 40 μm

2. Objective lenses with a higher NA and longer WD are desirable.

3. A femtosecond-pulsed infrared laser is also available from Spectra-Physics (MaiTai).

4. The dichroic and filter set required depends on the fluorescent proteins and dyes used.

5. We utilize a Carl Zeiss upright multiphoton microscope with internal 32-channel GaAsP spectral detectors when using simultaneous multiple fluorescent labels. This enables acquisition of the entire spectrum of each label in one scan, which is then used to create unmixed images.

6. The custom-made stereotactic stage is composed of a 10-mm-thick metal plate, on which two cylinders with screw holes are placed. The head holder can be fixed to this stage with two stainless screws.

7. The head holder has one recess, the curvature radius of which is 28 mm. The center of the recess has a hexagonal window. The head holder is 3 mm in thickness and 15 g in weight.

8. Some time is required for the laser and temperature to stabilize.

9. Remove as much hair as possible to prevent hair (which is autofluorescent) entering the visual field.

10. Prevent glue from contaminating the visual field because some glues are autofluorescent.

11. Do not fasten too tightly to avoid injuring the mouse.

12. The head holder is kept fully loaded with PBS by an infusion syringe pump.

13. The excitation wavelength of 940 nm is used to simultaneously excite ECFP, tdTomato, and pHocas-3. For an example of intravital time-lapse bone imaging, image stacks were collected at 3 μm vertical steps at a depth of 50–150 μm below the skull bone surface with 2.0× zoom, 512 × 512 X–Y resolution, and a time resolution of 5 min.

14. The heart rate is used as a guide to adjust the anesthetic gas concentration.

References

1. Hattner R, Epker BN, Frost HM (1965) Suggested sequential mode of control of changes in cell behavior in adult bone remodeling. Nature 206:489–490

2. Sims NA, Martin TJ (2014) Coupling the activities of bone formation and resorption: a multitude of signals within the basic multicellular unit. Bonekey Rep 3:481

3. Cahalan MD, Parker I, Wei SH, Miller MJ (2002) Two-photon tissue imaging: seeing the immune system in a fresh light. Nat Rev Immunol 2:872–880

4. Germain RN, Miller MJ, Dustin ML, Nussenzweig MC (2006) Dynamic imaging of the immune system: progress, pitfalls and promise. Nat Rev Immunol 6:497–507

5. Ishii M et al (2009) Sphingosine-1-phosphate mobilizes osteoclast precursors and regulates bone homeostasis. Nature 458:524–528

6. Ishii M, Kikuta J, Shimazu Y, Meier-Schellersheim M, Germain RN (2010) Chemorepulsion by blood S1P regulates osteoclast precursor mobilization and bone remodeling in vivo. J Exp Med 207:2793–2798

7. Kikuta J et al (2013) Sphingosine-1-phosphate-mediated osteoclast precursor monocyte migration is a critical point of control in the anti-bone-resorptive action of active vitamin D. Proc Natl Acad Sci U S A 110:7009–7013

8. Kikuta J et al (2013) Dynamic visualization of RANKL- and Th17-mediated osteoclast function. J Clin Invest 123:866–873

9. Kowada T et al (2011) *In vivo* fluorescence imaging of bone-resorbing osteoclasts. J Am Chem Soc 33:17772–17776

10. Maeda H et al (2016) Real-time intravital imaging of pH variation associated with osteoclast activity. Nat Chem Biol 12:579–585

11. Loudet A, Burgess K (2007) BODIPY dyes and their derivatives: syntheses and spectroscopic properties. Chem Rev 107:4891–4932

12. Kozloff KM, Volakis LI, Marini JC, Caird MS (2010) Near-infrared fluorescent probe traces bisphosphonate delivery and retention *in vivo*. J Bone Miner Res 25:1748–1758

Chapter 2

Intravital Imaging of Mouse Bone Marrow: Hemodynamics and Vascular Permeability

Yookyung Jung, Joel A. Spencer, Anthony P. Raphael, Juwell W. Wu, Clemens Alt, Judith R. Runnels, Briaira Geiger, and Charles P. Lin

Abstract

The bone marrow is a unique microenvironment where blood cells are produced and released into the circulation. At the top of the blood cell lineage are the hematopoietic stem cells (HSC), which are thought to reside in close association with the bone marrow vascular endothelial cells (Morrison and Scadden, Nature 505:327–334, 2014). Recent efforts at characterizing the HSC niche have prompted us to make close examinations of two distinct types of blood vessel in the bone marrow, the arteriolar vessels originating from arteries and sinusoidal vessels connected to veins. We found the two vessel types to exhibit different vascular permabilites, hemodynamics, cell trafficking behaviors, and oxygen content (Itkin et al., Nature 532:323–328, 2016; Spencer et al., Nature 508:269–273, 2014). Here, we describe a method to quantitatively measure the permeability and hemodynamics of arterioles and sinusoids in murine calvarial bone marrow using intravital microscopy.

Key words Bone marrow blood vessel, Arterioles, Sinusoids, Permeability, Hemodynamics, Flow speed, Blood vessel diameter, Mouse restraint, Intravital imaging

1 Introduction

The microanatomic landscape of the bone marrow is dominated by the presence of a dense vascular network. The vasculature makes up approximately 25–30% of the marrow space by volume [1, 2], with sinusoidal blood vessels being the most prominent vessel type. However, the bone marrow vasculature is heterogeneous [3, 4], and the heterogeneity is particularly notable when imaging the local hemodynamics in real time [1, 5]. Compared to arteriolar vessels, the flow speed and sheer rate in sinusoidal vessels are much lower [1, 5], and vascular permeability is significantly higher [5]. Increased vascular permeability has been shown to increase the level of reactive oxygen species (ROS) in the surrounding cells and

Yookyung Jung and Joel A. Spencer contributed equally to this work.

Masaru Ishii (ed.), *Intravital Imaging of Dynamic Bone and Immune Systems: Methods and Protocols*, Methods in Molecular Biology, vol. 1763, https://doi.org/10.1007/978-1-4939-7762-8_2, © Springer Science+Business Media, LLC 2018

to impact the migration and differentiation of hematopoietic stem and progenitor cells (HSPCs) [5]. Here, we present a protocol for measuring hemodynamics and permeability of arterioles and sinusoids in mouse bone marrow using video rate laser scanning confocal/two-photon microscopy [6–8]. Video rate laser scanning is achieved by a polygon-based fast scanning mechanism that allows full-frame (500 × 500 pixels) image acquisition at 30 frames per second. Higher frame rates can be acquired at a reduced frame size (120 frames per second at 500 × 125 pixels). The rapid scanning enables individual hemodynamic and vessel permeability measurements based on fluorescently labeled circulating blood cells and vascular dye leakage, respectively. Using this protocol, we could measure flow speeds up to 10 mm/s in individual blood vessels and simultaneously record vascular permeability in the same vessels within the first minute after dye injection. We also present concurrent methods for stabilizing the mouse for imaging and injection of cells and dyes on stage using a custom-built catheter.

2 Materials

2.1 Mouse

Any strain of mice can be used. Care should be taken to minimize signal overlap with the vascular dyes for permeability studies if co-injecting fluorescently labeled cells or using transgenic fluorescent mouse models. We typically use C57BL/6, which is the most common background strain for our studies. Animals were maintained in the animal facilities of Massachusetts General Hospital in compliance with institutional guidelines, and all animal studies were approved by the Subcommittee on Research Animal Care of the institution.

The high resolution imaging demands minimal mouse movement during imaging caused by breathing and other movement artifacts (*see* **Note 1**). Adequate mouse restraint can be achieved by modifying a 50 mL conical tube as described in [4]. However, with improved access to rapid-prototyping and related CAD software, more precise restraints can be fabricated. Our custom-built, 3D printed mouse restraint was designed using Autodesk® Inventor Professional 3D CAD software (Autodesk®, USA) and printed on a Fortus 380mc (Stratasys, USA) using ASA filament (*see* **Note 2**).

2.2 Fluorescence Labeling of Red Blood Cells (RBCs)

Fluorescently labeled RBCs are used for flow speed measurement. Here we assumed that the local blood flow speed is equal to the average speed of RBCs in the vasculature.

Solutions and heparin-coated microcentrifuge tubes should be prepared immediately before RBC labeling.

1. Fluorescent cell label CFDA-SE: thaw one vial of 500 μg CFDA-SE (V12883, Invitrogen) and solubilize in 90 μL DMSO.

2. Labeling solution A ("Soln A"): 90 mL of PBS (without calcium and magnesium) supplemented with 1 g/L glucose and 0.1% bovine serum albumin (BSA). Keep 60 mL at room temperature, warm 30 mL to 37 °C.

3. Labeling solution B ("Soln B"): 48 mL PBS (without calcium and magnesium), warm to 37 °C.

4. Wash solution ("Soln W"): 30 mL PBS (without calcium and magnesium) supplemented with 1 g/L glucose. Keep at room temperature.

5. Donor mouse: we label 1.2×10^9 RBCs for a final yield of $>0.75 \times 10^9$ cells. In our experience, a single facebleed from an adult unanesthetized C57BL/6 mouse provides sufficient RBCs.

6. Microcentrifuge tube for blood collection: add 200 μL 100 unit/mL heparin into tube and vortex briefly to coat.

7. Any BSA stock solution (concentration varies by manufacturer).

2.3 Fluorescence Labeling of the Vasculature

Vascular dyes are used for flow speed measurement, vessel diameter measurement, and vascular permeability measurement.

1. Large molecular weight fluorescent dye-dextran conjugates: 10 mg/mL 70 kDa Rhodamine B-dextran, 10 mg/mL 70 kDa Texas red-dextran, 10 mg/mL 70 kDa FITC-dextran.

2.4 Custom-Built Catheter

1. 30½ gauge needle.

2. Tygon microbore tubing, 0.010 (ID) × 0.030 (OD) in.

3. ½ cc insulin syringe with 29 G × ½ in. needle.

3 Methods

3.1 Preparing Fluorescently Labeled RBCs

RBCs are fluorescently labeled ex vivo and injected into recipient mouse 2–3 days before imaging to allow time for the bone marrow to re-establish its equilibrium hemodynamic state.

1. Perform facial vein blood collection on donor mouse and collect the blood in heparin-coated microcentrifuge tube. Animal anesthesia (if used) should be non-intravenous, such as isoflurane. Avoid ketamine and xylazine.

2. Transfer the heparinized blood suspension into 12 mL of Soln A at room temperature. Centrifuge at $500 \times g$ for 6 min. Discard the suspension, which should be opaque with a faint red shade. The cell pellet should be bright red.

3. Wash the RBCs two more times with 1.5 mL Soln A at room temperature.

4. Perform cell count. Resuspend 1.2×10^9 RBCs in 12 mL Soln A (37 °C) at 1×10^8 cells/mL. Keep the cells at 37 °C.

5. Add the 90 μL CFDA-SE DMSO stock into Soln B. Vortex to mix and split the solution evenly into two 50 mL centrifuge tubes (24 mL each).

6. Mix 6 mL of the RBC suspension from **step 4** into each of the two 50 mL centrifuge tubes prepared in **step 5**. Label at 37 °C for 12 min.

7. When labeling is complete, introduce bovine serum albumin stock solution such that BSA concentration is 0.1% in each of the two 50 mL centrifuge tubes. Centrifuge.

8. Wash each cell pellet in 30 mL Soln A at room temperature. Centrifuge.

9. Resuspend each cell pellet in 15 mL Soln W at room temperature and combine the two suspensions into one centrifuge tube. Perform cell count and centrifuge.

10. Resuspend the labeled RBCs in 180 μL saline for retro-orbital or tail vein injection. The RBC suspension should retain the same bright red hue as in blood; do not inject cells that look "rusty" as they will be cleared by circulation.

3.2 Mouse Restraint and Preparation

1. Anesthesia is induced using 4% isoflurane in oxygen with a maintenance rate of 1–3%. Induction is achieved in a separate chamber prior to mounting the mouse in the restraint.

2. For minimal motion, the mouse is first restrained by the bite-bar, followed by the nose cone and lastly the side skull restraints. The contact points on the side of the skull should be between the eye socket and ears, typically in the region of the squamosal bones (*see* Fig. 1).

3. Following appropriate restraint, the skull is prepared after scalp incision [7].

3.3 Intravital Imaging of Calvarial Bone Marrow

The protocol for performing intravital optical imaging of the bone marrow has been well described [6–8]. It is summarized as follows. Figure 2a shows the cross-sectional view of the calvarial bone of a mouse. As the bone overlying the marrow cavity is typically 50–70 μm thick, the bone marrow can be accessed optically after a simple skin flap surgery to expose the underlying bone surface. The thickness of the marrow cavity can vary from tens of micrometers to a couple of hundred micrometers (Fig. 2a and b), where the low intensity region in between the bone layers is the bone marrow. Using the intrinsic second harmonic signal to visualize

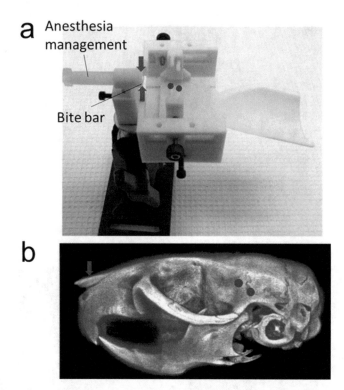

Fig. 1 3D printed mouse holder for intravital optical imaging. (**a**) Mouse holder. Red arrows indicate the nose cone and bite-bar which are anchor points for securing the mouse head. Red dots are prongs that fix squamosal bones of the mouse. (**b**) Side view of mouse skull. Red arrows and dots of (**a**) are shown at the corresponding sites [6]

the bone, we image the bone marrow cavities located in the central region of the skull around the sagittal and coronal sutures, which encompass an area approximately 3–6 by 6–8 mm (*see* Fig. 2c and **Note 3**). An example image of a bone marrow cavity of a nestin-GFP mouse is shown in Fig. 2d, with the bone signal in blue, GFP in green, hematopoietic stem and progenitor cell in red, and blood vessels in grey. The cell is overlaid on the pre-acquired nestin-GFP, blood vessels, and bone images.

3.4 Imaging Labeled RBC and Calculating Flow Speed

The blood flow speed is measured by tracking the frame-to-frame displacement of individual RBCs using high frame rate imaging. 750–800 million fluorescently labeled RBCs are injected into a recipient mouse 2–3 days before imaging. Immediately prior to imaging, a fluorescent vascular dye (e.g., Rhodamine-B-dextran) is injected allowing the visualization of the blood vessels that map the "paths" of RBC displacement. For accurate flow speed measurement, the average velocity of a minimum of five RBCs is used.

The detailed protocol for determining RBC and blood flow speed in vivo is as follows:

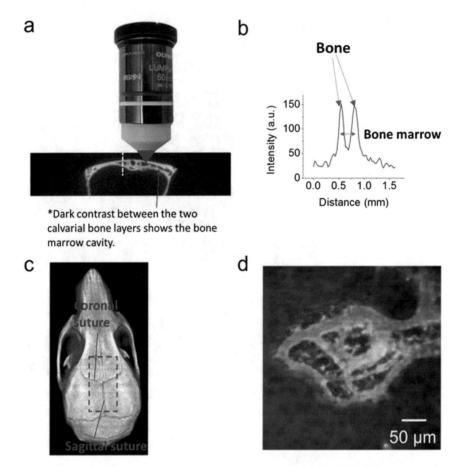

Fig. 2 Intravital optical imaging of the bone marrow through the calvarial bone. (**a**) Cross-sectional view of a mouse skull (from Henkelman M, Micro-CT images of mouse skull. http://www.stlfinder.com/model/mouse-skull-(from-micro-ct)) and optical access into the bone marrow between calvarial bone layers. (**b**) Intensity profile of the dotted yellow line in (**a**) shows two layers of calvarial bone and bone marrow between them. (**c**) Top view of a mouse skull. Optical imaging area is shown as a dotted red rectangle that contains coronal and sagittal sutures [6]. (**d**) Example of in vivo optical imaging of the bone marrow [9]. Nestin-GFP (green), hematopoietic stem and progenitor cell (red), blood vessels (grey), and bone (blue) are displayed. The cell is overlaid on the pre-acquired nestin-GFP, blood vessels, and bone images. Scale bar is 50 μm

1. Deliver 40 μL of 10 mg/mL 70 kDa Rhodamine B-dextran (ThermoFisher Scientific) to a labeled RBC recipient mouse by retro-orbital or tail vein intravenous (i.v.) injection for vascular labeling.

2. Perform simultaneous in vivo imaging of bone, blood vessels, and labeled RBC. Imaging conditions are as follows:

   - Image size: 500 × 125 pixels.

   - Imaging speed: 120 frames/s.

   - Bone: 840 nm femtosecond laser excitation, ~40 mW of power at the sample, 80 MHz repetition rate, MaiTai,

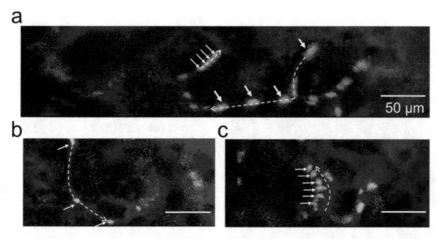

Fig. 3 Flow of labeled RBCs in the bone marrow blood vessels. Blue: second harmonic generation signal from bone collagen. Red: blood vessels. Green: labeled RBCs. Scale bars are 50 μm. (**a**) Example image showing overlay of labeled RBCs at several consecutive frames. (**b**) Flow of a single RBC in an arteriole. (**c**) Flow of a single RBC in a sinusoid

Spectra Physics, Collection of the second harmonic generation from collagen in bone.

- CFSE-labeled RBC: 491 nm continuous wave (CW) laser excitation, ~1 mW of power at the sample, Dual Calypso, Cobolt, Collection of confocal fluorescence at the spectral range of 509–547 nm.

- Blood vessel: 561 nm CW laser excitation, Jive, Cobolt, ~1 mW of power at the sample, Collection of confocal fluorescence at the spectral range of 573–613 nm.

3. Calculate the speed of the blood flow using the following equation (*see* **Note 4**):

    Total distance traveled by RBC/Time (= number of frames × 1/120 s).

The flow of labeled RBCs in the bone marrow blood vessels is shown (Fig. 3). The labeled RBCs at several consecutive frames are overlaid on the vascular image. Dotted and solid arrows show the direction of flow and the positions of RBCs at each frame, respectively.

Arterioles with small diameters (5–10 μm) show fast flow (>1.5 mm/s) (Fig. 3b), and sinusoids with large diameter (>20 μm) show slow flow (<1 mm/s) (Fig. 3c).

3.5 Blood Vessel Diameter Measurement

Based on the flow speed and vessel diameter (Fig. 4), the majority of bone marrow blood vessels can be categorized into two distinct groups (Fig. 4f), those with high flow speed and small diameter

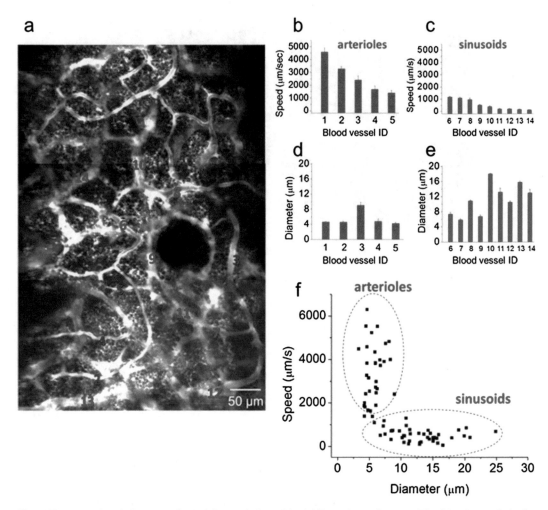

Fig. 4 Flow speed and diameter of arterioles and sinusoids. (**a**) Two-photon image of the blood vessels in the calvarial bone marrow. Numbers in red and blue indicate the blood vessel identification (ID). Scale bar is 50 μm. (**b, c**) Individual blood vessel flow speeds from arterioles and sinusoids, respectively. (**d, e**) Individual blood vessel diameters from arterioles and sinusoids, respectively. (**f**) Scatterplot of flow speed as a function of diameter. Two distinct groups of "high flow speed and small diameter" vs "low flow speed and large diameter" can be found (data from 70 blood vessels, $n = 6$ mice). Specific site of the individual blood vessels with ID numbers in (**b–e**) can be found in (**a**)

(arterioles) vs those with low flow speed and large diameter (sinusoids). These results are consistent with published values [1].

The protocol for blood vessel diameter measurement is as follows:

1. Deliver 40 μL of 10 mg/mL 70 kDa Rhodamine B-dextran (ThermoFisher Scientific) by retro-orbital or tail vein intravenous (i.v.) injection for vascular labeling.

2. Acquire two-photon excitation fluorescence (at the spectral range of 550–680 nm) image of the vessels in the calvarial bone marrow immediately after injecting the vascular dye with femto-

second laser source (~40 mW of power at the sample, 80 MHz repetition rate, 840 nm, MaiTai, Spectra Physics). Example image shown in Fig. 4a.

3. Measure the diameter of the blood vessels using image analysis software, for example ImageJ or Fiji software [10]. Repeated measurements are taken and the averaged value of the measured diameters is acquired.

3.6 Preparation of Custom-Built Catheter for Vascular Imaging and Permeability Measurement

Because of the high permeability of the bone marrow vasculature, it is necessary to perform dye injection while the mouse is on stage, so that the early dynamics of dye leakage immediately after injection can be recorded and analyzed.

3.6.1 Catheter Preparation

1. Cut 30½ gauge needle by using forceps (Fig. 5(1)).

2. Insert the cut needle into 0.030 in. flexible plastic tube (Fig. 5(2)).

3. Insert a needle of an insulin syringe into the other end of the plastic tube (Fig. 5(3)).

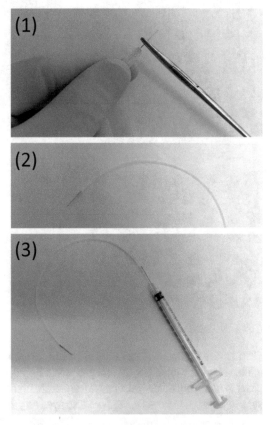

Fig. 5 Preparation of home-built catheter for repeated vascular imaging and permeability measurement

4. Repeated bone marrow vascular imaging and permeability measurements can be performed by using the home-built catheter.

5. In case multiple measurements of permeability are necessary, vasculature dyes with distinct two-photon emission spectrum should be used to prevent the signal leaking between the detection channels (*see* **Note 5**).

3.6.2 Quantitative Measurement of Permeability

1. Perform video rate two-photon imaging of bone marrow vasculature immediately after injection of vascular dye.

2. Frame-to-frame misalignment of the images can exist because of residual movement artifacts from breathing (Fig. 6a).

3. Series of raw images in Fig. 6a are registered and aligned by either using Template Matching plugin of ImageJ or Matlab code utilizing the command, normxcorr2, which performs normalized two-dimensional cross-correlation [11, 12]. Ten

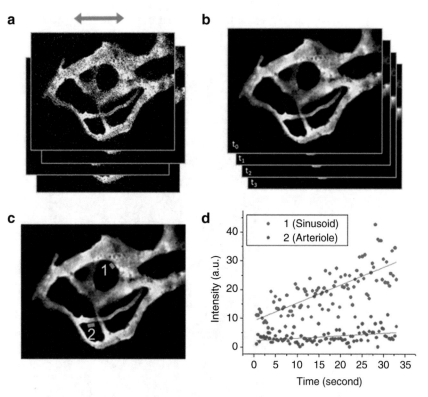

Fig. 6 Process to measure the rate of vascular dye leakage. (**a**) Series of two-photon raw vascular images with 1/30 s of time interval. Misalignment of the images exists because of residual movement artifacts. (**b**) Raw images are registered and aligned. Ten consecutive frames are frame-averaged to reduce the background noise signal. (**c**) Regions to measure the dye leakage are displayed as yellow rectangles labeled with 1 (next to sinusoid) and 2 (next to arteriole). (**d**) Average intensity in the region 1 and 2 of (**c**) is plotted as a function of time. The linear fits are shown as red lines. The slope of this linear fit is the rate of vascular dye leakage, dI/dt

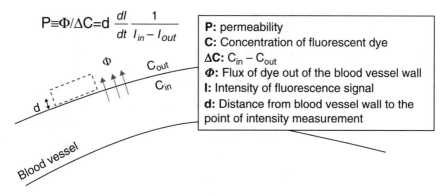

Fig. 7 Calculation of permeability by Fick's law of diffusion

consecutive frames are frame-averaged to reduce the background noise signal (Fig. 6b).

4. Select regions of interests (ROIs) to measure the rate of vascular dye leakage (Fig. 6c).

5. Plot the intensity measured from the ROIs as a function of time. Average intensity measured from region 1 and 2 in Fig. 6c is plotted in Fig. 6d.

6. The slope of the linear fit (solid red line in Fig. 6d) from "Intensity vs time" plot is the rate of vascular dye leakage, dI/dt.

7. Calculate the permeability value by equation based on Fick's law of diffusion [13] (*see* **Note 6**) (Fig. 7).

4   Notes

1. To minimize mouse motion, the restraint should at least consist of a: (1) bite-bar to fix the top jaw under the teeth; (2) nose cone to provide anesthesia and press down on the nasal bone; and (3) adjustable side skull support that can be firmly closed to accommodate different animal sizes.

2. Any 3D CAD software can be used if it can export stl files, which is the file format required by 3D printers. In relation to 3D printers, the majority of current benchtop models have tolerances within the 100–200 μm range suitable for printing a mouse restraint.

3. Imaging outside the dotted rectangle is also possible, but re-positioning of the mouse skull might be necessary because of the great curvature of the skull.

4. For accurate measurement of the total distance traveled by RBC, the length of the segmented line along the blood vessels is acquired using Fiji [10].

5. For multiple vascular imaging, the dye with longer emission spectrum should be used earlier than the one with shorter emission spectrum. This is because the dye spectra generally have long tails towards long wavelengths and the fluorescence of this spectral tail can leak into the other detection channel.

6. The d in the permeability equation is the distance between the blood vessel wall and the point of intensity measurement. Consecutive ROIs should be selected next to the vessel so that there are no gaps between them. A half thickness of ROI can be used as d in the permeability equation.

Acknowledgement

This work is supported in part by NIH grant EB017274, DK103074, and HL 095489 (to C.P.L.), by IBS-R023-Y1 (to Y.J.), and by the Australian National Health and Medical Research Council (NHMRC), Early Career Fellowship #APP1088318 (to A.P.R.).

References

1. Spencer JA, Ferraro F, Roussakis E et al (2014) Direct measurement of local oxygen concentration in the bone marrow of live animals. Nature 508:269–273

2. Kunisaki Y et al (2013) Arteriolar niches maintain haematopoietic stem cell quiescence. Nature 502:637–643

3. Nombela-Arrieta C et al (2013) Quantitative imaging of haematopoietic stem and progenitor cell localization and hypoxic status in the bone marrow microenvironment. Nat Cell Biol 15:533–543

4. Li XM, Hu Z, Jorgenson ML, Slayton WB (2009) High levels of acetylated low-density lipoprotein uptake and low tyrosine kinase with immunoglobulin and epidermal growth factor homology domains-2 (Tie2) promoter activity distinguish sinusoids from other vessel types in murine bone marrow. Circulation 120:1910–1918

5. Itkin T, Gur-Cohen S, Spencer JA et al (2016) Distinct bone marrow blood vessels differentially regulate haematopoiesis. Nature 532:323–328

6. Veilleux I, Spencer JA, Biss DP et al (2008) In vivo cell tracking with video rate multimodal-ity laser scanning microscopy. IEEE J Sel Top Quantum Electron 14:10–18

7. Lo Celso C, Lin CP, Scadden DT (2011) In vivo imaging of transplanted hematopoietic stem and progenitor cells in mouse calvarium bone marrow. Nat Protoc 6:1–14

8. Wu JW, Runnels JM, Lin CP (2014) Intravital imaging of hematopoietic stem cells in the mouse skull. Methods Mol Biol 1185:247–265

9. Morrison SJ, Scadden DT (2014) The bone marrow niche for haematopoietic stem cells. Nature 505:327–334

10. Schindelin J, Arganda-Carreras I, Frise E et al (2012) Fiji: an open-source platform for biological-image analysis. Nat Methods 9: 676–682

11. Tseng Q, Wang I, Duchemin-Pelletier E et al (2011) A new micropatterning method of soft substrates reveals that different tumorigenic signals can promote or reduce cell contraction levels. Lab Chip 11:2231

12. Schneider CA, Rasband WS, Eliceiri KW (2012) NIH image to ImageJ: 25 years of image analysis. Nat Methods 9:671–675

13. Berg HC (1993) Random walks in biology. Princeton University Press, Princeton

Chapter 3

Bone Imaging: Platelet Formation Dynamics

Asuka Sakata and Satoshi Nishimura

Abstract

Bone imaging using multiphoton microscopy enables dynamic observation of platelet formation in living animals. Two-photon excitation microscopy is superior to confocal microscopy as it enables deeper tissue penetration, efficient light detection, and reduced phototoxicity. Using this microscopy approach, thrombopoiesis by megakaryocytes is clearly visualized in the skull at significant depth from the surface. Here we describe our microscopy setup and dye recipe for visualization of bone marrow in the mouse skull.

Key words In vivo imaging, Bone marrow imaging, Platelet production, Multiphoton microscope

1 Introduction

Platelet production is a dynamic phenomenon occurring in the bone marrow and lung [1, 2]. Platelets are formed and released into the bloodstream by megakaryocytes. Because megakaryocytes are rare myeloid cells and are located deep inside the body, the analysis of platelet production has been difficult. After the cloning of thrombopoietin [3], numerous studies of thrombopoiesis have been performed using cultured megakaryocytes [4, 5]; however little is known about the process of this in the body. Recently, two-photon microscopy has emerged as a powerful tool for imaging inside the living body. Previous in situ imaging approaches, such as electron microscopy, only provide static images [6, 7], while two-photon microscopy can provide dynamic observation inside the bone marrow. Using this approach, both morphological and dynamic environmental information can be obtained, including shear stress and cell kinetics [8, 9]. Through the observation of mouse skull bone marrow, we have identified a novel mode of thrombopoiesis, named "megakaryocyte rupture" [10]. The microscopy settings and dye recipe to carry out this bone marrow imaging are described herein.

Masaru Ishii (ed.), *Intravital Imaging of Dynamic Bone and Immune Systems: Methods and Protocols*, Methods in Molecular Biology, vol. 1763, https://doi.org/10.1007/978-1-4939-7762-8_3, © Springer Science+Business Media, LLC 2018

2 Materials

2.1 Microscope

Multiphoton inverted microscope (A1 R MP, Nikon, Japan) with a GaAsP external high-sensitive detector (Nikon, Japan), a femtosecond laser (Chameleon Vision II, Coherent, USA), and an objective with 1.25 numerical aperture (CFI Apo Lamda S 40XWI, Nikon, Japan) (*see* **Note 1**).

2.2 Animal Heater

Microscope-stage automatic thermocontrol system (ThermoPlate/Olympus, TOKAI HIT, Japan) (*see* **Note 2**).

2.3 Microscope Imaging Software

NIS Elements Advanced Research (Nikon, Japan).

2.4 Cover Glass

24 × 60 mm cover glass with a thickness of 0.12–0.17 mm.

2.5 Animals

Wild-type mouse (C57BL/6), C57BL/6-Tg (CAG-EGFP), or C57BL/6-Tg (PF4 cre) × C57BL/6-Cg-Tg(CAG-floxed neo EGFP) (*see* **Note 3**).

2.6 Anesthetic

Urethane solution (100 mg/ml): weigh 4 g of urethane and dilute to 40 ml with saline. Store at room temperature in a sealable tube (*see* **Note 4**).

2.7 Dyes and Antibodies

1. Rhodamine B dextran solution (100 mg/ml) for plasma staining: weigh 1 g of Rhodamine B dextran and add 10 ml of saline. Divide into tubes and store at −30 °C; avoid repeated freeze-thaw cycles.

2. Hoechst 33342 (60 mg/ml) for nuclear staining: weigh 100 mg of Hoechst 33342 and add 1.7 ml of saline. Divide into tubes and store at −30 °C in the dark; avoid repeated freeze-thaw cycles (*see* **Note 5**).

3. Dylight 488-labeled rat antibody (0.2 mg/ml) against the glycoprotein Ib beta subunit of the murine platelet/megakaryocyte-specific glycoprotein Ib-V-IX complex diluted in phosphate buffered saline containing 0.2% bovine serum albumin (X488) (*see* **Note 3**).

2.8 Surgical Instruments

Small animal scissors and forceps. Braided silk.

3 Methods

3.1 Animal Preparation

1. Prior to initiation of the animal procedure, warm the mouse using an incandescent lamp. This step enables dye injection into the tail vein more easily.

2. Inject 50 μl of Rhodamine B solution and 50 μl of Hoechst 33342 solution (and 50 μl of X488 for wild-type mice) into

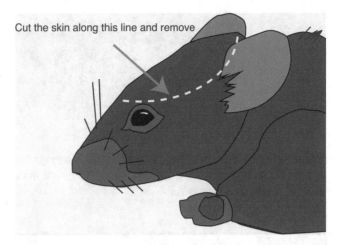

Fig. 1 Exposing the mouse skull. Grab the skin at the top of the mouse head with forceps. Using scissors, cut along the incision line shown in the figure

    the mouse through the tail vein using a 1 ml syringe and 30 G needle.

3. Inject 150 µl of urethane solution into the mouse peritoneum. Wait for 2–3 min then check the depth of anesthesia by clipping the paw with forceps. If the depth of anesthesia is shallow, add another 50 µl of urethane solution and check the depth again.

4. Remove the skin from the top of the head to expose the skull (Fig. 1).

3.2 Animal Fixation on the Stage (Fig. 2)

1. Place the cover glass just above the objective lens.

2. Turn the animal heater on and lay the mouse on the stage in a supine position.

3. Hold the mouse head on the cover glass using the following method. Pull the mouse incisive tooth with braided silk forward and downward, and then fix the braided silk to the stage with scotch tape. Avoid making gaps between the cover glass and the cranium to as great an extent as possible.

4. Fill the gaps between the cover glass and cranium with saline.

3.3 Bone Marrow Imaging by Microscope

1. Set the IR laser wavelength to around 860 nm then start the observation. Bone and collagen are visualized as blue (wavelength 430 nm) by second harmonic generation. Nuclei are also visualized as blue (wavelength 461 nm). Find the red color (wavelength 580 nm: bloodstream) and green color (wavelength 509 nm: cytoplasm) inside the bone.

2. Focus on a megakaryocyte: visualized as a bright green cell with a large nucleus. We can see the proplatelets inside the bloodstream near the megakaryocytes. Proplatelets have many bulges that are interconnected with a thin bridge of cytoplasm. Platelets are released from the nascent tips of the proplatelets (Fig. 3a–d).

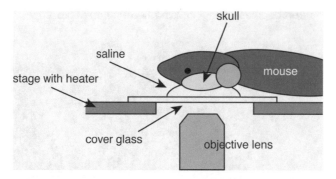

Fig. 2 Cover glass setup and animal fixation on the stage. Place the cover glass and mouse as shown in the figure. After fixation of the mouse head with braided silk hooked to the incisive tooth, fill the gap between the cover glass and mouse skull with saline

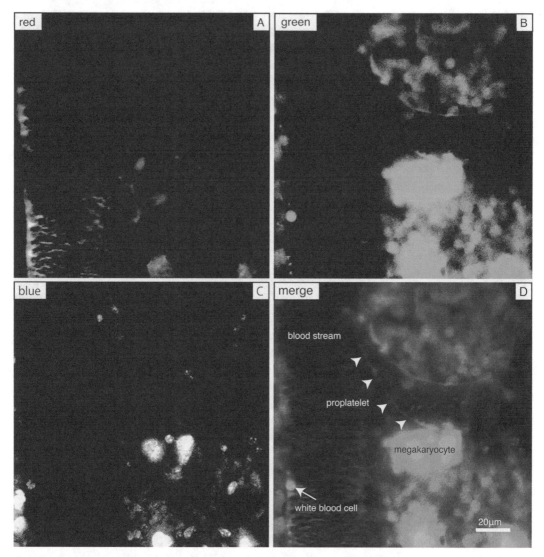

Fig. 3 Mouse skull bone marrow image. (**a**) Red; TRITC image, (**b**) Green; FITC image, (**c**) Blue; Hoechst image, and (**d**) merged image. A proplatelet elongated from the megakaryocyte is observed

4 Notes

1. Acquisition of bright, real-time, and long-duration movies deep inside the living body requires a microscope with a long-wavelength fast laser, a high-sensitive detector, and an objective with a large numerical aperture. The bone marrow observation can be carried out using an inverted or upright fluorescent microscope. An upright microscope allows the mouse to be easily set in the observation position and to remain upright; however, it is difficult to avoid distortion of the acquired image by respiratory movement. An inverted microscope can minimize breathing artifacts and compared with an upright microscope is relatively easy to make a wide perpendicular plane to the optical axis.

2. Hypothermia often leads to deterioration of the mouse general condition.

3. Mice <10 weeks old are better for bone imaging. When the C57BL/6-Tg(CAG-EGFP) mouse strain is used, we obtain brighter images compared with the other mouse strains. Using C57BL/6-Tg(PF4 cre) × C57BL/6-Cg-Tg(CAG-floxed neo EGFP) allows us to obtain platelet- and megakaryocyte-specific fluorescent images. The combination of using the wild-type mouse and X488 antibody (*see* Subheading 2.7, **item 3**) also provides platelet- and megakaryocyte-specific fluorescent images; however, the image is relatively dark.

4. Urethane has an oncogenic effect. Wear a mask and gloves when making the urethane solution. If possible, use the safety cabinet to avoid exposing urethane to co-workers. Add the saline gradually to the urethane when making the urethane solution. Add the saline up to a 40 ml solution: if a total of 40 ml of saline is added to the 4 g of urethane, the final volume of solution exceeds 40 ml considerably.

5. Hoechst 33342 is mutagenic. Wear a mask and gloves when making the Hoechst 33342 solution. If possible, use the safety cabinet to avoid exposing Hoechst 33342 to co-workers. When making the Hoechst 33342 solution, it is not necessary to dissolve the compound completely. The final solution is often opaque.

References

1. Wright JH (1906) The origin and nature of the blood plates. Boston Med Surg J 23:643–645

2. Lafrançais E, Ortiz-Muñoz G, Caudrillier A et al (2017) The lung is a site of platelet biogenesis and a reservoir for haematopoietic progenitors. Nature 544(7648):105–109

3. Vigon I, Mornon JP, Cocault L et al (1992) Molecular cloning and characterization of MPL, the human homolog of the v-mpl oncogene: identification of a member of the hematopoietic growth factor receptor superfamily. Proc Natl Acad Sci U S A 89(12):5640–5644

4. Choi ES, Nichol JL, Hokom MM et al (1995) Platelets generating in vitro from proplatelet-displaying human megakaryocytes are functional. Blood 85(2):402–413

5. Cramer EM, Norol F, Guichard J et al (1997) Ultrastructure of platelet formation by human megakaryocytes cultured with the Mpl ligand. Blood 89(7):2336–2346

6. Becker RP, De Bruyn PP (1976) The transmural passage of blood cells into myeloid sinusoids and the entry of platelets into the sinusoidal circulation; a scanning electron microscopic investigation. Am J Anat 145(2):183–205

7. Radley JM, Scurfield G (1980) The mechanism of platelet release. Blood 56(6):996–999

8. Mazo IB, Gutierrez-Ramos JC, Frenette PS et al (1998) Hematopoietic progenitor cell rolling in bone marrow microvessels: parallel contributions by endothelial selectins and vascular cell adhesion molecule 1. J Exp Med 188(3):465–474

9. Zhang J, Varas F, Stadtfeld M et al (2007) CD41-YFP mice allow in vivo labeling of megakaryocytic cells and reveal a subset of platelets hyperreactive to thrombin stimulation. Exp Hematol 35(3):490–499

10. Nishimura S, Nagasaki M, Kunishima S et al (2015) IL-1α induces thrombopoiesis through megakaryocyte rupture in response to acute platelet needs. J Cell Biol 209(3):453–466

Chapter 4

Live Imaging of Interstitial T Cell Migration Using Lymph Node Slices

Tomoya Katakai

Abstract

Live imaging using various microscopic technologies is an indispensable tool for investigating the dynamic nature of immune cells. One of the most powerful techniques is the two-photon laser-scanning microscopy (TP-LSM), which has various advantages in observing deep tissues in vivo. Interstitial T cell migration in the lymph node (LN) is a phenomenon intensively examined using TP-LSM in the field of immunology. Intravital and explant methods have been standards for imaging T cell behaviors in the LN, though there are several limitations. Live imaging of LN slices, an LN explant sliced by a vibratome to expose tissue parenchyma, could provide an alternative approach with technical advantages for an in-depth analysis of interstitial T cell migration in vivo.

Key words Interstitial migration, Lymph node, Tissue slice, T cells, Two-photon microscopy

1 Introduction

Efficient immune responses are accomplished by the orchestration of a variety of immune cells that are circulating and actively moving within their internal environment. Live imaging utilizing various microscopic technologies is therefore an indispensable tool for understanding the mechanisms underlying such a dynamic nature of immune system. One of the most powerful techniques is the two-photon laser-scanning microscopy (TP-LSM) [1–3]. Near-infrared femtosecond pulse-laser is used as the light source to allow for the various advantages of the TP-LSM; it allows for excitation of fluorescent materials present deep inside of tissues and for detection of signals with a high spatial resolution. Since two-photon excitation occurs only at the focus, stacks of optical slices can be obtained to enable the reconstruction of three-dimensional (3D) views. Two-photon excitation using near-infrared light also reduces phototoxicity, owing to the generation of reactive oxygen species that causes cellular damages and inhibits motility, especially in actively migrating cells.

Masaru Ishii (ed.), *Intravital Imaging of Dynamic Bone and Immune Systems: Methods and Protocols*, Methods in Molecular Biology, vol. 1763, https://doi.org/10.1007/978-1-4939-7762-8_4, © Springer Science+Business Media, LLC 2018

One of the first applications of live imaging using TP-LSM to the immune system was for observing the behavior of lymphocytes in the lymph node (LN), which clearly demonstrated a surprisingly dynamic migration of lymphocytes in a densely packed interstitial environment [4]. In particular, T cells show remarkably high-speed migrations at average velocities of more than 10 μm/min. At present, intranodal lymphocyte migration is one of the best-examined live behaviors of immune cells [5–18]. Intravital and explant methods are commonly used for LN imaging [2, 19]. Intravital imaging is performed on surgically exposed LNs in anesthetized animals, in which the local temperature and moisture are carefully maintained [6, 8, 20, 21]. This allows for an accurate reflection of physiological conditions owing to the preservation of blood and lymph supplies; however, surgical operations and vital conditioning of animals under anesthesia require special skills and devices. In contrast, the explant method involves the examination on isolated LNs under the perfusion of a warm and oxygen-saturated medium, and it is technically easier than the intravital method [4, 5, 9]. Although the LNs are isolated from blood and lymph circulations, lymphocyte migration in explanted LNs is known to be comparable to that in intravital imaging.

To visualize the interstitial migration of T cells in the LN, fluorescently labeled cells that have been injected intravenously and entered the LNs are often examined [1, 4]. In this setting, the injected lymphocytes that are circulating in the blood need to pass though high endothelial venules (HEVs), which act as a barrier to the LN, to approach the tissue parenchyma [22, 23]. Lymphocytes isolated from genetically modified mice are also used to analyze molecular functions. However, this remains a problem associated with passage through the HEV barrier; some of the molecular machineries required for interstitial migration (chemokines, adhesion molecules, signaling pathways, and cytoskeletal dynamics for motility) are likely to be shared by the process for passage through the HEVs [17, 18, 24–27]. Therefore, defects in these molecular components could diminish the efficiency of lymphocyte entry into the LN before reaching the parenchyma, whereas cells that are still capable of entering the tissue in such a condition are possibly enriched with a biased population containing certain specific characteristics. The administration of antibodies or drugs for in vivo suppression can potentially cause similar problems. In addition, in vivo treatments require a relatively large amount of reagents and raise concerns about the kinetics and delivery to the target tissues. Moreover, even in TP-LSM, live imaging through the LN capsule with sufficient resolutions can be applied at most 200–300 μm below the surface. Thus, the deeper parts or the center of the LN are out of examination range.

Utilizing LN tissue slices present a potential to circumvent these problems [28–31]. With the use of a vibratome, isolated LNs are sliced to expose the deeper parts of the tissue. This method is capable of allowing lymphocytes from the section surface to penetrate the tissue parenchyma directly, although lymphocytes that have entered the tissue by adoptive transfer can also be examined. In addition, migration of normal lymphocyte can be modulated immediately by adding small amounts of antibodies or drugs. Because of its broad potential applications, LN slices are useful for investigating lymphocyte behaviors and dynamics in a three-dimensional (3D) tissue environment.

In this chapter, preparation of LN slices and T lymphocytes for visualizing interstitial motility is described in detail. The success or failure of experiments largely depends on the careful handling and manipulation of tissues and cells. However, procedures of TP-LSM are not described in detail, since they are similar to the standard methods of explant imaging as described in previous studies [9, 29, 32], and because the settings and operations of the microscopes and devices differ from system to system.

2 Materials

1. Plastic coverslips.
2. Instant adhesive: Aron Alpha/Krazy Glue.
3. Low gelling temperature (LGT) agarose: Agarose type VII-A.
4. Phosphate buffered saline (PBS).
5. Cell preparation medium (CPM): RPMI 1640 supplemented with 1% fetal calf serum (FCS) and 10 mM HEPES.
6. Magnetic cell sorting reagents: MACS® Pan T cell isolation kit II, mouse.
7. Magnetic cell sorter: MidiMACS™ separator.
8. Magnetic cell sorting column: MACS® LS columns.
9. Orange fluorescent dye: CellTracker™ Orange, CMTMR ((5-(and-6)-(((4-chloromethyl) benzoyl amino) tetramethyl-rhodamine)) (Excitation/Emission Max.: 541/565 nm), 1 mM in DMSO.
10. Green fluorescent dye: CellTrace™ CFSE, CFSE (5-(and-6)-Carboxyfluorescein Diacetate, Succinimidyl Ester) (Excitation/Emission max: 492/517 nm), 1 mM in DMSO.
11. Tissue adhesive: Vetbond™ (3M Animal Care Products).
12. Vibrating microtome (vibratome): Linear slicer Pro10.
13. Double edge razor blade.
14. Acetone.
15. Grease: High vacuum grease.
16. Perfusion medium: RPMI 1640 medium.

3 Methods

3.1 Making the Plastic Pedestal for the LNs

A small pedestal with a suitable shape that is easy to handle is required for the stabilization of the LN onto it for slicing, transport, and placement in the perfusion chamber. A handmade plastic pedestal is shown here.

1. Prepare the pieces of plastic coverslips by cutting the original size into 8 × 8 mm (1) and 4 × 4 mm (2) using scissors (Fig. 1a).

2. Make small pieces of plastic blocks by cutting a conventionally used flat-bottom plastic culture dish into 2 × 2 mm (3) (Fig. 1a). First, make long rectangular pieces (~4 mm in width) by a cutter, subsequently cut them into smaller pieces (2 × 4 mm) by a nipper, and finally make small cubic pieces (2 × 2 mm).

3. Assemble the parts into a pedestal, in the order of (1), (3), and (2) from the bottom using instant adhesive as shown in Fig. 1b and c.

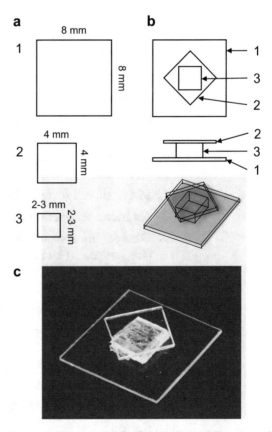

Fig. 1 The handmade plastic pedestal for the LN slice. (**a**) The sizes of the components made from plastic coverslips (1 and 2) or a dish (3). (**b**) Assembly of the parts to make the pedestal. (**c**) Photograph of the pedestal

3.2 Preparation of 4% LGT Agarose-PBS Gel Solution

To cut a soft and small LN, the whole organ needs to be covered with a supportive gel. LGT agarose is hardened below 37 °C, which allows the LN to be embedded in the gel without exposure to high temperatures.

1. Measure 4 g LGT agarose powder and 100 mL PBS into a 300 mL conical flask.

2. Dissolve agarose in PBS in a microwave oven (*see* **Note 1**).

3. After the agarose is completely dissolved, seal the flask mouth using a wrap film and keep warm in a water bath at 50 °C. The flask should be moved to 37 °C shortly before use (*see* Subheading 3.7, **step 1**). For storage of the remaining agarose gel, *see* **Note 2**.

3.3 Isolation of LNs

One of the advantages of the LN slice method is the ability for multiple examinations using different parameters in a single experiment via multiple LNs. For this purpose, LNs are isolated from a mouse and stored at room temperature (RT).

1. Prepare a medium for tissue or cell preparation (CPM) (*see* **Note 3**).

2. Dispense 1 mL CPM into Eppendorf tubes for the required number of LN slices. Label the name of LN on the cap.

3. Carefully remove the superficial LNs (inguinal, brachial, axillary, and cervical) from a mouse, trying not to damage the organs (*see* **Note 4**). Put a pair of LNs (left and right) into one Eppendorf tube with CPM. The LNs are stored at RT until use (during the preparation of T cells).

3.4 Preparation of T Cells by Magnetic Sorting

T cells are isolated from secondary lymphoid tissues such as the LNs and spleen by several methods. Magnetic cell sorting (MACS) is used here with some modification. Removing unnecessary cells for enriching the desired cell population, i.e., cells with no antibody bound (negative selection), is more preferable. Using freshly prepared CPM is critical for T cell isolation.

1. Put a sterilized stainless mesh and 5 mL CPM in a culture dish.

2. Remove the remaining LNs and/or the spleen from the same mouse above or additional LNs from another mouse (depending on the number of cells required) and place them in the dish.

3. Mash the organs on the stainless mesh with forceps and pipette the released cells for several times to make a single cell suspension (*see* **Note 5**).

4. Collect the cell suspension to a 15 mL tube and centrifuge it at $300 \times g$ at RT for 4 min.

5. Discard the supernatant, add fresh 5 mL CPM, and suspend the cells. Determine the recovered cell number by cell counting or measuring the concentration.

6. Centrifugation; 1300 rpm, RT, 4 min.

7. Discard the supernatant, add 0.1–0.3 mL CPM (depending on the cell number), and resuspend it.

8. Label the cells with the antibody cocktail and with the microbeads from the MACS® Pan T cell isolation kit. The amounts of antibody cocktail and microbeads solution are determined according to the manufacturer's instruction.

9. Add 5 mL CPM and vortex it. Centrifugation; 1300 rpm, RT, 4 min.

10. During the centrifugation, set up the MACS® separator apparatus; attach a LS column to the separator magnet on support and place a 15 mL tube under the column for cell collection. Pass 2 mL CPM through the column in advance.

11. After centrifugation, remove the supernatant, add fresh 0.5–1 mL CPM, and suspend the cells.

12. Add the cell suspension to the column.

13. After the cell suspension has entered the column, add 2 mL CPM (first wash).

14. After the medium has entered the column, add 2 mL CPM again (second wash).

15. Centrifuge the collection tube; 1300 rpm, RT, 4 min.

16. Discard the supernatant, add 1 mL CPM, and resuspend the cells. Determine the recovered cell number.

3.5 Fluorescent Labeling of T Cells

Fluorescent labeling of lymphocytes with CMTMR or CFSE is frequently used for visualizing cell motility in live imaging because of their high labeling efficiency, brightness, sustainability, and low toxicity in optimal labeling concentrations. This step is not required if the cells already expressing fluorescent proteins are used.

1. Prepare a ~1 × 10^7 cells/mL T cell suspension in CPM in a 15 mL tube.

2. Add the CMTMR (final 5 μM) or CFSE (final 2 μM) solution and mix quickly. Incubate the cells at 37 °C, for 20–30 min and keep protected from light. During this step, LNs are adhered to the pedestal.

3. Add 5 mL CPM and mix by vortex mixer. Centrifugation; 1300 rpm, RT, 4 min.

4. Discard the supernatant, add fresh 5 mL CPM, and resuspend the cells. Centrifugation; 1300 rpm, RT, 4 min.

5. Repeat **step 4**.

6. Discard the supernatant, add fresh CPM for a final concentration of 1×10^6 cells/100 μL, and suspend the cells using P1000 micropipette.

7. Incubate at 37 °C in a CO_2 incubator until use.

3.6 Adhesion of the LN to the Pedestal

1. Take the LNs out of tubes and put them into a medium (1:1 CPM:PBS) in a dish.

2. Carefully remove adipose tissues as well as the blood and lymphatic vessels that are attached to the LNs using fine-tip forceps and a Vannas-style spring scissor under a binocular microscope (*see* **Note 6**). Operate all the LNs before proceeding to **step 3**.

3. Put a small amount of Vetbond™ tissue adhesive (<0.2 μL) on the center of the handmade pedestal. Spread the adhesive to the size of the LN and blot up the excess through the edge of a small piece of Kimwipe (*see* **Note 7**).

4. Place a LN on a Kimwipe and wipe off the surface medium by gentle rolling, in particular with respect to the medullary side.

5. Put the LN in the center of pedestal with the cortical side upward (Fig. 2a and h) and carefully push the top of the LN using forceps.

6. Soak the LN/pedestal quickly into CPM/PBS solution and coagulate Vetbond™. If some bubbles of the polymer are formed, remove them with forceps.

7. Return the LN/pedestal to the same Eppendorf tube.

8. Repeat the **steps 3–7** for all LNs.

3.7 Embedding of LN in LGT Agarose Gel

All the LNs on the pedestal are embedded in agarose gel in this part.

1. Move the 4% LGT agarose solution in the conical flask from the 50 °C to a 37 °C water bath that is close to the work space. Cut 5 mm off a P1000 micropipette tip.

2. Take all the LN/pedestals out from their tubes and align them on an extended Kimwipe to remove medium from the bottom of the pedestals. Be sure to discriminate each LN.

3. Remove medium from the lower part (on the lower plate) of the pedestals with Kimwipes, but keep the upper parts of the pedestals wet (i.e., LNs).

4. Move the LN/pedestal and align them again on a flat black table or bench. A black bench makes it easier to see the gel. Be sure to identify each LN.

5. Remove medium from the upper part with a Kimwipe. Wipe medium off the surface of the LN carefully and do it for all LNs as quickly as possible.

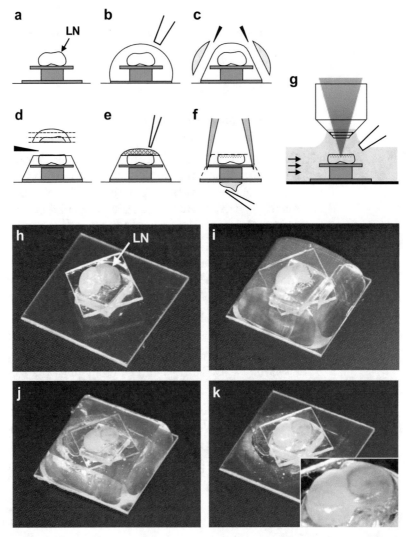

Fig. 2 Procedure for producing LN slices. (**a**–**g**) Schematic representation for each step. The LN is adhered to the pedestal (**a**), embedding in LGT agarose gel (**b**), trimming the four sides gel droplet (**c**), cutting the LN via a vibratome (**d**), loading the T cell suspension onto the section (**e**), removing the gel, carrying the LN/pedestal by thin tip forceps, and putting the grease on the bottom (**f**), and placing it in the perfusion chamber (**g**). (**h**–**k**) Photographs of the procedure. Each photograph (**h**), (**i**), (**j**), and (**k**) corresponds to (**a**), (**c**), (**d**), and (**f**), respectively. Inset in (**k**) shows a higher magnification of the LN slice

6. Take 4% LGT agarose with the cut P1000 micropipette; try not to get any air bubbles into the gel solution. Pour the gel slowly onto the lower part of the pedestal first and subsequently on the upper part to cover whole LN (Fig. 2b) (*see* **Note 8**). Repeat for all LNs as quickly as possible.

7. After the gel is solidified for a few minutes, remove the four sides of the swelled gel parts with a cutter to make a dome-and-pyramid shape (Fig. 2c and i).

8. Return them to the same Eppendorf tubes.

3.8 LN Slicing and T Cell Loading onto the Sections

Cutting the LN using a vibratome and loading the lymphocytes onto the sections are processes that require the most skillful technique, since it could affect the results of the examination. All the steps need to be done quickly and smoothly.

1. Put the required number of T cells into an Eppendorf tube that has been coated with CPM, which has removed before use (*see* **Note 9**). Place at 37 °C in a CO_2 incubator until **step 11** of Subheading 3.8. If the pretreatment of antibodies or drugs is required, add them at this step.

2. Soak a laser blade in a small amount of acetone to remove the oil coat. Wipe the oil and acetone off and dry well. Set the blade on the vibratome.

3. Put 0.2–0.5 μL of the instant adhesive onto the center of sample tray.

4. Take one LN/pedestal embedded in agarose gel from its tube and wipe the medium off the bottom of pedestal. Adhere the LN/pedestal to the center of sample tray (*see* **Note 10**).

5. Set the sample tray onto the microtome and move the height of tray to a position so that the blade is slightly higher than the LN.

6. Pour PBS into the tray so that the gel is completely soaked.

7. Start cutting from the top of the gel in the following settings (in the case of Linear Slicer Pro10): amplitude 0.5–1 mm, frequency 81–82 Hz, and step 300 μm. Set the speed of blade feeding adequately for cutting the gel part.

8. Repeat gel cutting until the blade is near the top of the LN. Carefully control the height of the blade by changing steps to a position where the blade finally skims over or slightly cut the top of the LN surface (Fig. 2d).

9. Determine the next step size of the blade between 200–300 μm, depending on the thickness of the first section and the size of the LN (*see* **Note 11**).

10. Cut the LN. Just before the blade is about to enter the tissue, reduce the speed of blade feed to 3–4 mm/min, and proceed to slicing (Fig. 2d and j) (*see* **Note 12**).

11. Centrifuge the lymphocytes in the tube prepared above (**step 1** of Subheading 3.8). For immediate inhibition experiments, add antibodies or drugs before this centrifugation.

12. Discard the supernatant, leaving 10–15 μL medium, and place the tube in the incubator.

13. Insert flat forceps between the sample tray and the pedestal to detach the pedestal from the tray. Carry the LN/pedestal with flat forceps.

14. Put the sliced LN/pedestal on a Kimwipe to remove liquids from the four sides of the gel.

15. Resuspend the cells and load the suspension onto the section (Fig. 2e) (*see* **Note 13**).

16. Incubate the LN slice at 37 °C in a CO_2 incubator for 30 min (*see* **Note 14**).

3.9 Setting of LN Slice in Perfusion Chamber

1. Remove the gel from the LN/pedestal by making a small cut and splitting with forceps without touching the LN (Fig. 2f and k).

2. Carry the LN/pedestal to the microscope by holding the upper plate of the pedestal using thin tip forceps (Fig. 2f). Put grease to the bottom of pedestal (Fig. 2f) and adhere onto the bottom of perfusion chamber by pushing the pedestal (Fig. 2g). Microscope and perfusion system are prepared in advance and warmed-up until this step.

3. Adjust the volume of the medium in the chamber by changing the suction rate of waste so that the LN slice is covered with the medium (Fig. 2g).

4. Adjust the lens to medium and focus onto the surface of LN slice under bright field.

5. Check for two-photon signals from the cells that accumulated on the LN slice surface. Remove excess cells from the surface by gently flashing the medium with a P1000 micropipette (Fig. 2g) (*see* **Note 15**).

3.10 Outline of Perfusion and Examination by TP-LSM

A heated chamber and peristaltic perfusion system is set up on the stage of the microscope. Warm RPMI 1640 medium saturated with 95% O_2 and 5% CO_2 via bubbling is sent to the chamber by a peristaltic pump at 2 mL/min. The temperature of medium in the chamber is adjusted to 36.5 ± 0.5 °C using a water bath, inline heater, and chamber heater. Z-stack images starting from 20–30 μm below the section surface are acquired using an 800–820 nm excitation wavelength. Typically, time-lapse images at 20 s interval for a duration of 20–30 min are obtained once or twice for each LN slice. Four-dimensional (x, y, z, t) image data sets are analyzed on Imaris or Volocity software (*see* **Notes 16** and **17**).

4 Notes

1. Since a 4% LGT agarose solution exhibits a high viscosity and may be boiled suddenly during microwave heating, careful dissolving/melting is required. To prevent bumping, pause the microwave frequently just before the agarose solution comes to a boil, stir it well, and heat again. Repeat this until all the agarose granules are dissolved.

2. After use, the remaining agarose solution is hardened at room temperature; the flask mouth is sealed with wrap film, and stored at 4 °C. This can be reused repeatedly, but repeated melting cycles may promote the evaporation of water from the gel and increase the concentration of agarose. In that case, add an appropriate volume of water, which will depend on the viscosity.

3. CPM must be freshly prepared in every experiment. For this, small aliquots (~1 mL) of FCS are cryopreserved. Do not use culture media containing FCS that have been preserved at 4 °C for long periods, because lymphocytes prepared in such stored media often show a reduced motility for unknown reasons.

4. Try to take the LN by picking up adipose or connective tissues and avoid directly touching LN as much as possible. Attachment of some adipose tissues is not problematic at this stage. Taking the LN accompanied with surrounding adipose tissue would be safe for beginners to keep the LN intact. The adipose tissues will be removed later (*see* the **step 2** of Subheading 3.6). If necessary, other LNs, such as popliteal and mesenteric LNs, can be used for tissue slicing.

5. The preparation of lymphocytes from lymphoid tissues is performed by reseachers' own ways. To maintain the ability of lymphocyte migration, the whole process should be performed at room temperature. Do not put the cells at 4 °C.

6. Do not make injuries in the LN. Operate as quickly as possible. It is sufficient to remove most of the appendages.

7. Vetbond rapidly coagulates in the presence of water. Using a micropipette (P2), minimally coat the surface with <0.2 μL vetbond. If vetbond is used in excess, the surface of the LN may be extensively covered with the coagulated vetbond polymer.

8. If the amount of gel poured is adequate, it will form a dome-like shape (Fig. 2b). Excess amount of gel may flow out of the pedestal; in that case, add additional gel.

9. For a standard analysis of normal T cell migration, $2–5 \times 10^5$ cells are required for each LN slice. Increased number of cells may be required for some inhibitory experiments or if the cells are from genetically modified mice due to a reduced motility. To minimize the loss of cells by adsorption to the inner surface of plastic tube, tubes should be filled with CPM in advance to be coated with FCS proteins.

10. The part of the LN that is to be examined should be placed on the opposite side of the blade entrance, because the tissue may be broken if the blade does not enter smoothly.

11. A smaller step size (thickness of a slice) below 100 μm may not make for good slices.

12. The blade angle to the surface of the LN is important for success of the initial blade entry. A smaller angle may cause a failure of blade entry, which could damage the tissue. Fine and flat sections are critical to allow for efficient entry of lymphocytes.

13. Applying the cell suspension in a volume greater than 15 μL may cause overflow and a loss of the suspension from the top of the LN/gel surface. In such a case, recover the cell suspension as much as possible, remove wetness from the sides of gel, and apply the cell suspension again. If the gel has a crack, the cell suspension will fall. In that case, use another LN slice.

14. Incubation for a longer period may cause the surface of the LN slice to dry. Medium should be added to maintain moisture.

15. If excess cells are present on the section, the fluorescent signals from the inside will be significantly reduced. Removing the excess cells will improve the signal. Sliced LNs will be expanded slightly for about 10 min after soaking in warm perfusion medium, therefore the focus will change.

16. The LN tissues and lymphocytes are steadily degraded, reducing viability and activity over time after removal from the body. Interstitial T cell migration also shows a tendency to decrease gradually. Therefore, comparing the data obtained at early and late time points on the same day may not be suitable for quantitative analysis. We typically compare a pair of image data obtained successively or in close periods.

17. During live imaging, cell behaviors often differ between every image field even in the same tissue, organ, or individual animal under the same experimental condition. Therefore, some researchers emphasize the importance of comparing phenomena within the same image, especially for quantitative analysis. The average velocity of interstitial T cell migration may also change from image to image. Thus, comparing two cell populations with different characteristics or genetic backgrounds in the same image is ideal. However, this is a strong limitation for the comparative analysis of various conditions. Even though the data sets are derived from different images, reproducibility of the experimental observations increases the reliability of the results. In fact, by taking advantage of LN slice examination to compare multiple parameters in the repetition of experiments, we were able to obtain results with clear significance (see Ref. [29–31]).

Acknowledgements

This work was supported by a Grant-in-Aid for Scientific Research on Innovative Areas (24111005) from The Ministry of Education, Culture, Sports, Science and Technology of Japan.

References

1. Cahalan MD, Parker I, Wei SH, Miller MJ (2002) Two-photon tissue imaging: seeing the immune system in a fresh light. Nat Rev Immunol 2:872–880

2. Germain RN, Miller MJ, Dustin ML, Nussenzweig MC (2006) Dynamic imaging of the immune system: progress, pitfalls and promise. Nat Rev Immunol 6:497–507

3. Bullen A, Friedman RS, Krummel MF (2009) Two-photon imaging of the immune system: a custom technology platform for high-speed, multicolor tissue imaging of immune responses. Curr Top Microbiol Immunol 334:1–29

4. Miller MJ, Wei SH, Parker I, Cahalan MD (2002) Two-photon imaging of lymphocyte motility and antigen response in intact lymph node. Science 296:1869–1873

5. Bousso P, Robey E (2003) Dynamics of CD8+ T cell priming by dendritic cells in intact lymph nodes. Nat Immunol 4:579–585

6. Miller MJ, Wei SH, Cahalan MD, Parker I (2003) Autonomous T cell trafficking examined in vivo with intravital two-photon microscopy. Proc Natl Acad Sci U S A 100:2604–2609

7. Miller MJ, Safrina O, Parker I, Cahalan MD (2004) Imaging the single cell dynamics of CD4+ T cell activation by dendritic cells in lymph nodes. J Exp Med 200:847–856

8. Mempel TR, Henrickson SE, Von Andrian UH (2004) T-cell priming by dendritic cells in lymph nodes occurs in three distinct phases. Nature 427:154–159

9. Okada T et al (2005) Antigen-engaged B cells undergo chemotaxis toward the T zone and form motile conjugates with helper T cells. PLoS Biol 3:e150

10. Woolf E et al (2007) Lymph node chemokines promote sustained T lymphocyte motility without triggering stable integrin adhesiveness in the absence of shear forces. Nat Immunol 8:1076–1085

11. Worbs T, Mempel TR, Bolter J, von Andrian UH, Forster R (2007) CCR7 ligands stimulate the intranodal motility of T lymphocytes in vivo. J Exp Med 204:489–495

12. Nombela-Arrieta C et al (2007) A central role for DOCK2 during interstitial lymphocyte motility and sphingosine-1-phosphate-mediated egress. J Exp Med 204:497–510

13. Okada T, Cyster JG (2007) CC chemokine receptor 7 contributes to Gi-dependent T cell motility in the lymph node. J Immunol 178: 2973–2978

14. Huang JH et al (2007) Requirements for T lymphocyte migration in explanted lymph nodes. J Immunol 178:7747–7755

15. Allen CD, Okada T, Tang HL, Cyster JG (2007) Imaging of germinal center selection events during affinity maturation. Science 315: 528–531

16. Cahalan MD, Parker I (2008) Choreography of cell motility and interaction dynamics imaged by two-photon microscopy in lymphoid organs. Annu Rev Immunol 26:585–626

17. Okada T (2010) Two-photon microscopy analysis of leukocyte trafficking and motility. Semin Immunopathol 32:215–225

18. Munoz MA, Biro M, Weninger W (2014) T cell migration in intact lymph nodes in vivo. Curr Opin Cell Biol 30:17–24

19. Cahalan MD, Parker I (2006) Imaging the choreography of lymphocyte trafficking and the immune response. Curr Opin Immunol 18:476–482

20. Mempel TR, Scimone ML, Mora JR, von Andrian UH (2004) In vivo imaging of leukocyte trafficking in blood vessels and tissues. Curr Opin Immunol 16:406–417

21. Sumen C, Mempel TR, Mazo IB, von Andrian UH (2004) Intravital microscopy: visualizing immunity in context. Immunity 21:315–329

22. von Andrian UH, Mempel TR (2003) Homing and cellular traffic in lymph nodes. Nat Rev Immunol 3:867–878

23. Miyasaka M, Tanaka T (2004) Lymphocyte trafficking across high endothelial venules: dogmas and enigmas. Nat Rev Immunol 4:360–370

24. Friedl P, Weigelin B (2008) Interstitial leukocyte migration and immune function. Nat Immunol 9:960–969

25. Kinashi T (2005) Intracellular signalling controlling integrin activation in lymphocytes. Nat Rev Immunol 5:546–559

26. Hogg N, Laschinger M, Giles K, McDowall A (2003) T-cell integrins: more than just sticking points. J Cell Sci 116:4695–4705

27. Lammermann T, Germain RN (2014) The multiple faces of leukocyte interstitial migration. Semin Immunopathol 36:227–251

28. Asperti-Boursin F, Real E, Bismuth G, Trautmann A, Donnadieu E (2007) CCR7 ligands control basal T cell motility within lymph node slices in a phosphoinositide 3-kinase-independent manner. J Exp Med 204:1167–1179

29. Katakai T, Habiro K, Kinashi T (2013) Dendritic cells regulate high-speed interstitial T cell migration in the lymph node via LFA-1/ICAM-1. J Immunol 191:1188–1199

30. Katakai T, Kondo N, Ueda Y, Kinashi T (2014) Autotaxin produced by stromal cells promotes LFA-1-independent and Rho-dependent interstitial T cell motility in the lymph node paracortex. J Immunol 193:617–626

31. Katakai T, Kinashi T (2016) Microenvironmental control of high-speed interstitial T cell migration in the lymph node. Front Immunol 7:194

32. Katagiri K et al (2009) Mst1 controls lymphocyte trafficking and interstitial motility within lymph nodes. EMBO J 28:1319–1331

Chapter 5

Two-Photon Imaging of T-Cell Motility in Lymph Nodes: In Vivo and Ex Vivo Approaches

Akira Takeda, Masayuki Miyasaka, and Eiji Umemoto

Abstract

T-cell motility is essential for the T cells' ability to scan antigens within lymph nodes and initiate contact with antigen-presenting cells. While T-cell migration has been extensively studied using in vitro migration assays, accumulating evidence indicates that the T-cell migration within lymph nodes is modulated by the surrounding cells and extracellular matrix, which form the confined architecture of the lymph nodes. Therefore, to understand the mechanisms of T-cell motility in vivo, their cell migration must be analyzed under physiological conditions. To this end, two-photon microscopy is extremely useful; this technique enables the tracking of fluorescently labeled cells in vivo and ex vivo, with high spatial and temporal resolutions. Here we describe the experimental procedures for applying two-photon microscopy to the in vivo and ex vivo imaging of T-cell migration in mouse lymph nodes. These approaches provide physiological insight into the mechanisms of T-cell behavior at a single-cell level in the three-dimensional lymph node environment.

Key words Two-photon microscopy, T-cell motility, Imaging

---

1 Introduction

Lymph nodes (LNs) are organs within which immune responses are initiated. T cells migrate from the blood to LNs through high endothelial venules, and then migrate continuously along the fibroblastic reticular cell (FRC) network in the LNs [1] where they scan antigens presented by antigen-presenting cells such as dendritic cells. The communication between T cells and antigen-presenting cells is an early step in adaptive immunity, triggering either a positive immune response or tolerance. Therefore, T-cell migration within the LNs is indispensable for immune induction. Recent studies showed that the T-cell motility within LNs is regulated by FRCs, which produce IL-7 [2] and CCL19 [3], and by the highly cell-dense structure of LNs [4, 5]. While T cells closely interact with FRCs, they do not require integrin-dependent signaling for their migration in the cell-dense three-dimensional

Masaru Ishii (ed.), *Intravital Imaging of Dynamic Bone and Immune Systems: Methods and Protocols*, Methods in Molecular Biology, vol. 1763, https://doi.org/10.1007/978-1-4939-7762-8_5, © Springer Science+Business Media, LLC 2018

environment of LNs, in contrast to their movement on two-dimensional matrix substrates [6], and this integrin-independent T-cell migration in LNs is at least partially regulated by FRC-produced lipid mediators such as lysophosphatidic acid [4, 7]. These studies emphasize the importance of studying T-cell migration within LNs under physiological conditions.

Two-photon microscopy is often used to track the migration of fluorescently labeled cells within tissues, including LNs. Excitation with two photons enables the photons to penetrate deep into intact tissues, and the use of photons with longer wavelengths helps to minimize photodamage and bleaching in tissues. These advantages of two-photon microscopy permit the monitoring of leukocyte migration in intact tissues in a physiologically relevant manner.

Here we describe two experimental procedures for tracing intranodal T-cell behavior using two-photon microscopy, i.e., for in vivo and ex vivo imaging. For in vivo imaging, we mainly use popliteal LNs, because they are easily accessible from the skin surface, and the adipose tissue enwrapping the LNs is relatively limited. Furthermore, blood vessels and lymphatics entering and leaving the node can be visualized relatively easily, so the popliteal LNs are particularly suitable for analyzing T-cell migration through the blood vessels and lymphatics. On the other hand, ex vivo analysis is performed using explanted LNs set in a flow chamber. This approach does not require the specialized instruments or microsurgical techniques needed for in vivo imaging. The cell movement in explanted LNs is reported to be comparable to that in vivo [8], although caution is necessary for data interpretation, since the perfusion medium does not perfectly mimic the blood and lymph flow. These in vivo and ex vivo approaches offer high resolution and sensitivity due to a lack of movement artifacts, and therefore have experimental advantages for deciphering the mechanisms of T-cell motility. They are also suitable for assessing the effect of gene deficiencies or pharmacological inhibition on T-cell motility in a physiological context.

2   Materials

2.1   Preparation of Donor T Cells

1. Six- to 12-week-old mice.

2. Immunomagnetic negative selection kit for CD4$^+$ or CD8$^+$ T cells.

3. Cell tracker dye: 5-(and -6-)-(((4-chloromethyl)benzoyl) amino) tetramethylrhodamine (CMTMR) or 5-(6)-carboxyfluorescein diacetate succinimidyl ester (CFSE).

4. RPMI1640 supplemented with 2% FCS.

2.2 Preparation of a Mouse Stage for In Vivo Imaging	1. 100-mm glass Petri dish (e.g., from Corning).
	2. 100-mm plastic Petri dish (e.g., from Corning).
	3. Superglue.
	4. Two lids of PCR tubes.

2.3 Surgical Anesthesia

1. Medetomidine.
2. Butorphanol.
3. Midazolam.
4. Phosphate-buffered saline (PBS) without $MgCl_2$ or $CaCl_2$.

2.4 Microsurgical Preparation of Mouse Popliteal LNs

1. Hair removal cream.
2. Electric trimmer.
3. Tissue adhesive.
4. PBS.
5. Heating pad.
6. Fine tweezers (Dumont #5).
7. Vannas spring scissors.

2.5 Preparation of LN Explants in a Flow Chamber

1. Flow chamber (custom-made).
2. Water bath.
3. RPMI1640 without phenol red.
4. Tygon tubing.
5. Two peristaltic pumps.
6. Tissue adhesive.
7. 35-mm glass-bottom dish.
8. Plastic coverslip.
9. Carbogen (95% oxygen/5% carbon dioxide)
10. Probe thermometer.

2.6 In Vivo or Ex Vivo two-Photon Imaging

1. Upright two-photon microscope equipped with non-descanned photomultiplier tube (PMT) detectors (e.g., TCS SP5, Leica), a high numerical aperture (N.A.) water immersion objective (e.g., HCX APO, 20x, N.A. 1.0, Leica), and a femtosecond-pulsed infrared laser (e.g., MaiTai Ti: sapphire-pulsed laser, Spectra-Physics).

2. Heating pad equipped with a temperature controller and a rectal probe (e.g., model HP-1 M, TCAT-2LV, and RET-3, respectively, Braintree Scientific, Inc.).

3. Water bath.

2.7 Quantitative Analysis of T-Cell Migration

1. Image analysis software (e.g., Imaris, Bitplane; Volocity, PerkinElmer).

3 Methods

3.1 Adoptive Transfer of T Cells

1. Dissect the LNs and/or spleen from donor mice. Mechanically dissociate the tissues, and lyse red blood cells when the spleen is used. Isolate T cells using an immunomagnetic negative selection kit.

2. Incubate the isolated cells with 5 μM CMTMR or another cell tracker dye (e.g., CFSE) in RMPI1640 supplemented with 2% FCS for 20 min at 37 °C (*see* **Note 1**). Wash the cells twice and suspend them in PBS at 5×10^6 cells/200 μl. Intravenously inject 200 μl of the cell suspension into recipient mice.

3.2 Preparation of a Mouse Stage for In Vivo LN Imaging

Cut away a portion of a 100-mm plastic dish to make a crescent shape (Fig. 1b). Smooth the cut edge. Affix the cut dish to the edge of the glass Petri dish using superglue (Fig. 1b). Glue the lids of two domed-cap PCR tubes to the glass dish to anchor skin flaps.

3.3 Anesthesia and Surgery

1. One day after the donor cell transfer, anesthetize recipient mice by intraperitoneal injection of a mixture of medetomidine (0.3 mg/kg), butorphanol (5 mg/kg), midazolam (4 mg/kg), and PBS (*see* **Note 2**). If necessary, insert a 30 G needle connected to a piece of PE-10 polyethylene tubing (Becton Dickinson) into a tail vein to intravenously inject reagents (e.g., fluorescently labeled dextran) or cells during imaging (*see* **Note 3**). Make sure the mouse is fully anesthetized, by a lack of response to toe and tail pinches. Use an electric trimmer to cut hair on the right hind leg. Remove loose hair and apply hair removal cream to the shaved area. After a few minutes of application, remove the cream and clean the exposed skin with a wet paper towel.

2. During the surgery, maintain the body temperature using a heating pad. Place the mouse onto the holder, with the back of the right knee facing up (Fig. 1c). Secure the right toe to the edge of the glass Petri dish (Fig. 1c). Tape the arms, and stretch and tape the left leg to the upper dish of the holder. After fixing the mouse in position, place the holder under the dissection microscope. Using Vannas spring scissors, make an incision in the skin from the middle of the right leg up to the thigh. Make horizontal skin incisions at the top of the vertical incision to make skin flaps (Fig. 1d). Pull and fix both skin flaps to the PCR tube lids with tissue adhesive (Fig. 1e). The popliteal LNs within the popliteal fossa should be exposed very carefully. Remove surrounding adipose tissue and muscles from the

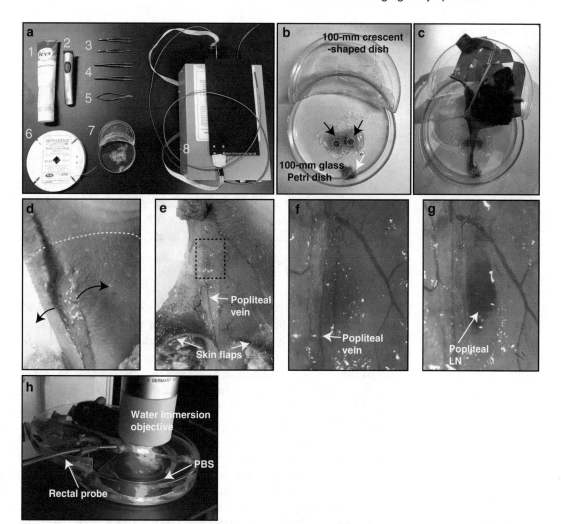

Fig. 1 Equipment and procedures for in vivo imaging of popliteal LNs. (**a**) 1: Hair removal cream; 2: Electronic trimmer; 3: Tweezers; 4: Fine tweezers (Dumont #5); 5: Vannas spring scissors; 6: catheter; 7: mouse holder; 8: rectal probe and temperature controller. (**b, c**) Mouse holder for in vivo imaging. A 100-mm crescent-shaped plastic dish is secured to a 100-mm glass Petri dish. The mouse's right leg is secured to the bottom of the glass dish (white arrow), and skin flaps are attached to the lids of PCR tubes (black arrows). (**d**) Zoom-in image of the leg area in (**c**). A horizontal incision is made near the top of the vertical incision, to create skin flaps at both sides. (**e**) Secure the skin flaps to the skin flap holders (**b**, black arrows). A LN is found alongside the popliteal vein. (**f**) Zoom-in image of the box in (**e**). The LN is dimly seen under muscle and adipose tissues. (**g**) Exposed LN. (**h**) After exposing the LN, the mouse is placed under the objective with a rectal probe. PBS is added to the bottom dish

popliteal LN using micro-dissecting tweezers (Dumont #5) (Fig. 1f and g). Expose the popliteal LN without affecting the integrity of the afferent and efferent blood vessels and the afferent lymphatic vessels (*see* **Notes 4** and **5**). After exposing the LN, insert a rectal feedback probe to maintain the body temperature at 37 °C (Fig. 1h) (*see* **Note 6**).

3.4 In Vivo two-Photon Microscopy of Popliteal LNs

1. Once the LN is exposed, immediately transfer the mouse holder to the two-photon microscope stage (Fig. 1h). Apply pre-warmed sterile PBS to the dish and make sure that the LN is submerged in PBS.

2. Set the temperature control to 37 °C and wait for the body temperature to increase. Use an epi-fluorescent lamp to place the popliteal LN under the objective. LNs can be found easily by searching for an accumulation of transferred cells. To track high-speed T-cell movement, imaging with a resonant scanner is recommended, because it enables images to be captured at a high frame rate. Acquire image stacks with appropriate time intervals (Fig. 3a). To track T-cell migration, acquire more than 30 x–y stacks spaced at 2–3 µm every 20–30 s.

3. After the imaging experiment, euthanize the animal by following an approved euthanasia protocol.

3.5 Setting up a Flow Chamber System for Ex Vivo Imaging

Warm the phenol red-free medium in a water bath at 40 °C and bubble a mixture of 95% O_2 and 5% CO_2 with a gas dispersion tube in the medium. Connect a reservoir for medium to a custom-built flow chamber (Fig. 2b) with Tygon tubing through a peristaltic pump (Fig. 2a). Warm the incoming medium and the flow chamber with heaters. In our custom-built chamber, the flow chamber is heated by circulating warmed water (Fig. 2b). Drain the medium from the chamber by connecting the flow chamber with a waste reservoir through the second peristaltic pump. The flow rate of medium through the chamber is regulated by the rotational speed of the two peristaltic pumps, which ideally should have the same speed. Continuously monitor the temperature of the medium in the flow chamber with a thermometer. Adjust the heaters or the water bath to obtain 37 °C in the flow chamber (approximately 40 °C in the water bath). Make sure that there are no air bubbles in the tubing and that the temperature in the flow chamber is stable.

3.6 Preparation of Explanted LNs

1. One day after donor cell injection, carefully dissect inguinal LNs using fine tweezers. Make sure that the LNs are not damaged; loss of integrity of the LN capsule affects the T-cell migration in LNs. If necessary, carefully remove the remaining fat from the LNs with fine tweezers under a dissecting microscope. The fat reduces the quality of the images because it scatters the light.

2. Secure the LNs to a plastic coverslip with a small amount of a tissue adhesive, which is applied to the coverslip beforehand. Secure the coverslip to a 35-mm dish by placing silicone grease on the bottom of the coverslip.

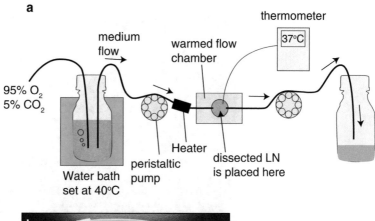

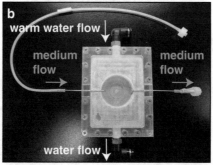

Fig. 2 Ex vivo imaging of LNs. (**a**) Perfusion system for ex vivo imaging. A dissected LN is placed in a flow chamber, and the medium, bubbled with a mixture of O_2 and CO_2, is continuously poured into and drained from the flow chamber. The medium flow is regulated by peristaltic pumps. The medium in the flow chamber is maintained at 37 °C by a water bath and by heating the incoming tubing. (**b**) Flow chamber used for an ex vivo imaging system. A 35-mm dish attached to a dissected LN is placed in the center of the flow chamber. Warmed medium is poured in and drained out as indicated. The temperature of the chamber is maintained by circulating warm water

3.7 Ex Vivo two-Photon Microscopy of Explanted LNs

Immediately after preparing the explanted LNs, set the 35-mm dish into the flow chamber. Make sure that the temperature in the chamber is around 37 °C (*see* **Note 7**). Place the flow chamber on the stage of a two-photon microscope, guide the LN under the objective using an epi-fluorescent lamp, and immediately start imaging as described in the in vivo imaging section (Subheading 3.4).

3.8 Data Analysis of In Vivo and Ex Vivo Two-Photon Imaging

Analyze the acquired time-lapse imaging stacks with image analysis software. To track T-cell migration, use the automated cell-tracking function of the software (Fig. 3b). The automatic mode is definitely helpful, but it cannot track the cells perfectly because of irregular T-cell migration movements within the LN (squeezing and jumping). Review the tracking made by the software and manually modify it (Fig. 3c) (*see* **Note 8**).

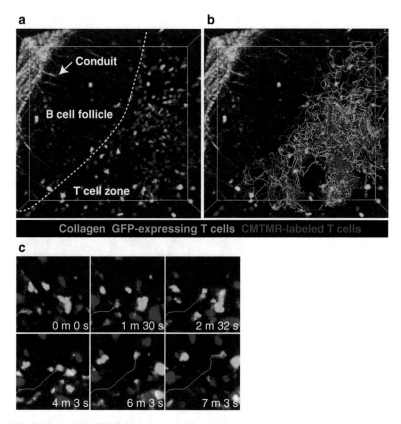

Fig. 3 Examples of LN imaging by two-photon microscopy. (**a**, **b**) In vivo two-photon imaging of T-cell migration in LNs. GFP-expressing T cells were mixed with an equal number of T cells labeled with CMTMR, and injected into a wild-type mouse. Collagen was visualized by second-harmonic generation imaging. The migration path of T cells was visualized in (**b**) using automated cell tracking. (**c**) Single T-cell tracking

Once the cell tracking is done, the *x*, *y*, *z* coordinates of T cells are automatically calculated by the software. Cell motility is analyzed by several parameters, including the cell velocity, directionality of cell motion, mean displacement, and motility coefficient [9]. The mean displacement (*D*) is the average distance after a certain time interval (*t*) and is plotted versus $t^{1/2}$ (mean displacement plot). The motility coefficient (*M*) is the volume in which an average cell can scan per unit time, and is calculated as $M = D^2/6t$. Mean displacement plots allow the type of cell migration to be identified (e.g., directional, random, or confined migration). Measure the cell velocity with the image analysis software. Import the *x*, *y*, *z* coordinates into the Excel software, and manually calculate the directionality of cell motion by dividing the net displacement by the total path length using >10-min tracks. Generate a mean displacement plot using the >10-min tracks by plotting the displacement *D*, which is calculated from the x, y, z coordinates of the cells, versus $t^{1/2}$, and calculate the motility coefficient as $M = D^2/6t$.

4 Notes

1. The use of transgenic fluorescent reporter animals (e.g., CAG-EGFP, DsRed) is recommended, because cell labeling with chemical reagents may affect the cell migration ability. Supplementation with a low concentration of FCS (1–2%) in the labeling buffer may help to maintain the cell migration ability. Perform preliminary experiments to make sure the cell labeling does not affect cell motility.

2. The effect of the anesthesia lasts for about 3 h. If the mouse wakes up during the imaging, subcutaneously inject the mixture again in a low dose.

3. To inject reagents to visualize the blood vasculature (e.g., fluorescently labeled dextran) or antibodies (e.g., anti-LFA1) during imaging, insert a 30 G needle connected to a piece of PE-10 polyethylene tubing before securing the mouse to the holder.

4. Intravital imaging is difficult and requires expertise in microsurgical procedures. Practice the surgery well before the experiment. Carefully determine the location of the popliteal LNs before exposing them. In young mice, the popliteal LNs are dimly visible after the skin incision. To visualize the LNs and afferent lymphatics, injecting Evans blue into the footpad is helpful. Note that Evans blue fluorescence (excitation at 620 nm, emission at 680 nm) is visualized by two-photon microscopy. Carefully expose the popliteal LNs without damaging the blood vessels and afferent lymphatics. The lymph flow from the afferent lymphatics is critical for observing the proper intranodal T-cell motility.

5. The use of young mice is recommended because old animals have more fat around the LNs than young ones, making it difficult to expose the popliteal LNs without damaging the surrounding blood vessels and lymphatics.

6. Keep the mouse's body temperature around 37 °C during the intravital imaging, because the T-cell motility in LNs depends on the temperature [10].

7. Carefully check the temperature in the flow chamber and the perfusion rate in ex vivo imaging. These factors strongly affect the T-cell motility in the explanted LNs [10].

8. The tracking of T-cell migration with image analysis software is time-consuming. Automated cell tracking is not perfect, and it is necessary to manually modify the cell-tracking results one by

one because of irregular T-cell migration. The use of a low amount of donor cells is also helpful for increasing the accuracy of automated tracking.

Acknowledgements

We thank Mr. Keita Aoi and Prof. Masaru Ishii (Osaka University) for their helpful advice in establishing procedures for the two-photon imaging of LNs.

References

1. Bajenoff M, Egen JG, Koo LY, Laugier JP, Brau F, Glaichenhaus N, Germain RN (2006) Stromal cell networks regulate lymphocyte entry, migration, and territoriality in lymph nodes. Immunity 25(6):989–1001. https://doi.org/10.1016/j.immuni.2006.10.011

2. Link A, Vogt TK, Favre S, Britschgi MR, Acha-Orbea H, Hinz B, Cyster JG, Luther SA (2007) Fibroblastic reticular cells in lymph nodes regulate the homeostasis of naive T cells. Nat Immunol 8(11):1255–1265. https://doi.org/10.1038/ni1513

3. Worbs T, Mempel TR, Bolter J, von Andrian UH, Forster R (2007) CCR7 ligands stimulate the intranodal motility of T lymphocytes in vivo. J Exp Med 204(3):489–495. https://doi.org/10.1084/jem.20061706

4. Takeda A, Kobayashi D, Aoi K, Sasaki N, Sugiura Y, Igarashi H, Tohya K, Inoue A, Hata E, Akahoshi N, Hayasaka H, Kikuta J, Scandella E, Ludewig B, Ishii S, Aoki J, Suematsu M, Ishii M, Takeda K, Jalkanen S, Miyasaka M, Umemoto E (2016) Fibroblastic reticular cell-derived lysophosphatidic acid regulates confined intranodal T-cell motility. eLife 5:e10561. https://doi.org/10.7554/eLife.10561

5. Jacobelli J, Friedman RS, Conti MA, Lennon-Dumenil AM, Piel M, Sorensen CM, Adelstein RS, Krummel MF (2010) Confinement-optimized three-dimensional T cell amoeboid motility is modulated via myosin IIA-regulated adhesions. Nat Immunol 11(10):953–961. https://doi.org/10.1038/ni.1936

6. Woolf E, Grigorova I, Sagiv A, Grabovsky V, Feigelson SW, Shulman Z, Hartmann T, Sixt M, Cyster JG, Alon R (2007) Lymph node chemokines promote sustained T lymphocyte motility without triggering stable integrin adhesiveness in the absence of shear forces. Nat Immunol 8(10):1076–1085. https://doi.org/10.1038/ni1499

7. Katakai T, Kondo N, Ueda Y, Kinashi T (2014) Autotaxin produced by stromal cells promotes LFA-1-independent and Rho-dependent interstitial T cell motility in the lymph node paracortex. J Immunol 193(2):617–626. https://doi.org/10.4049/jimmunol.1400565

8. Allen CD, Okada T, Tang HL, Cyster JG (2007) Imaging of germinal center selection events during affinity maturation. Science 315(5811):528–531. https://doi.org/10.1126/science.1136736

9. Sumen C, Mempel TR, Mazo IB, von Andrian UH (2004) Intravital microscopy: visualizing immunity in context. Immunity 21(3):315–329. https://doi.org/10.1016/j.immuni.2004.08.006

10. Huang JH, Cardenas-Navia LI, Caldwell CC, Plumb TJ, Radu CG, Rocha PN, Wilder T, Bromberg JS, Cronstein BN, Sitkovsky M, Dewhirst MW, Dustin ML (2007) Requirements for T lymphocyte migration in explanted lymph nodes. J Immunol 178(12):7747–7755

Chapter 6

Imaging the Lymph Node Stroma

Clément Ghigo, Rebecca Gentek, and Marc Bajénoff

Abstract

Lymph node (LN) stromal cells are being recognized as key organizers of the immune system. They assemble in complex 3D networks and hence, need to be studied in situ to fully understand their exact functions. Here, we describe two distinct but complementary procedures that allow analyzing LN stromal cells at high resolution by confocal imaging.

Key words Confocal imaging, Lymph node, Stroma, Cryostat sectioning, Vibratome sectioning, 3D reconstruction

1 Introduction

As the major sites of lymphocyte recirculation, lymph nodes (LN) play central roles in immunity. It is now increasingly acknowledged that stromal cells not only create the architecture of LN, but also actively control the function and survival of lymphocytes [1].

Despite this growing appreciation of their diverse functions, our understanding of LN stromal cell biology is still rather limited. Their exact developmental origin, organization, and functional dynamics have remained largely enigmatic, which is at least partially attributable to technical limitations: LN stromal cells are relatively rare, fragile cells that lose phenotypic and functional characteristics upon in vitro culture [2]. Therefore, solely relying on isolating stromal cells from LN and studying them ex vivo likely introduces experimental bias and yields flawed results. Although generally true for immune cells, this is particularly critical for LN stromal cells, whose function can only fully be appreciated within the intricate, dynamic network they form. Thus, in situ studies are key to study the biology of LN stromal cells. However, imaging of the LN stroma imposes specific challenges: While conventional confocal imaging approaches can achieve cellular resolution, the

---

Clément Ghigo and Rebecca Gentek contributed equally to this work

Masaru Ishii (ed.), *Intravital Imaging of Dynamic Bone and Immune Systems: Methods and Protocols*, Methods in Molecular Biology, vol. 1763, https://doi.org/10.1007/978-1-4939-7762-8_6, © Springer Science+Business Media, LLC 2018

tissue sections are too thin (8–30 μm) to analyze the complex 3D network of stromal cells. On the other hand, alternative imaging techniques such as Optical Projection Tomography (OPT) generally do not reach cellular resolution [3].

To overcome this hurdle, we describe here two distinct procedures to image LN stromal cell networks at high resolution by confocal imaging: (1) a cryostat-based method optimized for LN stromal cells and (2) a novel approach in which thick (200 μm) sections obtained with a vibratome can be optically clarified [4–8], enabling the reconstruction of a 3D network from acquired single images.

Given their characteristic features, we believe that the two imaging approaches described herein are complementary and instrumental to further elucidating the function and dynamics of LN stromal cells and their interactions with immune cells. Notably, both methods are compatible with endogenous fluorescent reporters and hence, can be combined for example with genetic fate mapping models.

Moreover, although originally established for imaging the LN stroma, we have since applied these techniques to a large variety of murine tissues across developmental stages. Thus, despite our initial focus, the methods described herein are more generally applicable to a broad spectrum of immunological and non-immunological questions and hence, provide a valuable resource even beyond the field of stromal cell biology.

2 Materials

Unless otherwise specified, reagents are handled and stored at room temperature (RT).

2.1 Common Materials for Cryostat and Vibratome Sectioning

1. Horizontal shaking platform (standard laboratory equipment).

2. Vacuum pump (standard laboratory equipment).

3. Tris buffer (1 M): To prepare 2 L of *stock* solution, dissolve 242.28 g of ultrapure Tris in 1.5 L of deionized water. Adjust the pH to 7.4 with HCl (about 150 ml) and fill up to a final volume of 2 L with deionized water. Dilute to obtain a 0.1 M *working solution*. Store at RT.

4. Immunohistochemistry (IHC) buffer: 0.5% w/v BSA and 2% v/v Triton X-100 in 0.1 M Tris buffer. Dissolve well. Store at 4 °C.

5. Primary and secondary antibodies targeting antigens of interest.

2.2 Materials for Cryostat Sectioning

1. Polystyrene tubes with screw caps.

2. Antigenfix reagent. Adhere to institutional guidelines for disposal of formaldehyde containing solutions.

3. Phosphate buffer: Dissolve 3.11 g of NaH_2PO_4 ($1H_2O$) and 11 g of Na_2HPO_4 (anhydrous) in deionized water. pH should be 7.4. Store at 4 °C.

4. Cryostat.

5. Sucrose solution (30%): Prepare a solution of 30% w/v sucrose in phosphate buffer. Filter using bottletop filter, keep sterile and store at 4 °C.

6. Tissue freezing medium (TFM) (Electron Microscopy Sciences).

7. Histology molds (Leica, reference 14702218311).

8. Superfrost plus adhesive microscope slides.

9. Hydrophobic glue pen.

10. Moisture staining chambers for microscopy slides.

11. Staining jars for microscopy slides.

12. Mounting medium.

2.3 Materials for Vibratome Sectioning

1. Thermoshaker for reaction tubes (standard laboratory equipment).

2. Agarose solution (4%): Add 4% w/v of low gelling temperature agarose to PBS. Bring to 70 °C to dissolve agarose powder. We recommend to prepare aliquots of 1 ml and store them at 4 °C.

3. Scalpel blades.

4. Superglue.

5. Vibratome.

6. 24 well tissue culture plates.

7. Clearing medium Rapiclear 1.47®.

3   Methods

3.1 Cryostat Sectioning

1. Carefully harvest the LN and transfer them to polystyrene tubes containing 3 ml of Antigenfix solution (*see* **Note 1**).

2. Fix the LN for 1 h at 4 °C under gentle agitation (*see* **Note 2**).

3. Remove the Antigenfix solution under a chemical hood (use proper disposal containers as Antigenfix is a PFA-based fixative).

4. Wash the LN in 3 ml phosphate buffer for 30 min to 1 h under gentle agitation at 4 °C.

5. Remove the phosphate buffer.

6. Dehydrate the samples in 3 ml sucrose solution overnight at 4 °C (*see* **Note 3**).

7. Fill the histology molds with TFM and embed the LN (*see* **Notes 4–6**) (Fig. 1).

8. Freeze the samples at −80 °C (*see* **Note 7**).

9. Remove the TFM-embedded sample blocks from histology molds (*see* **Note 8**).

10. Cut 25–50 µm thick LN slices using a cryostat. Set chamber temperature to −22 °C and object temperature to −23 °C.

11. Upon cutting, immediately transfer the tissue sections to Superfrost plus adhesive microscopy slides (*see* **Note 9**).

12. All the subsequent staining procedures are performed in moisture staining chambers protected from light.

13. Surround the sectioned tissues with a water-repellent barrier (hydrophobic pen).

14. Rehydrate the tissues by carefully adding 100–200 µl of Tris buffer directly onto the tissue sections (*see* **Note 10**) and incubate for 10 min. This step will also remove TFM (Fig. 2).

15. To remove Tris buffer, flip the slide and allow the solution to drain by gravity. Carefully remove any remaining buffer with an absorbent tissue (Fig. 3).

16. Add 100–200 µl of IHC buffer per tissue section and incubate for 20 min.

17. Remove the IHC buffer as described in **step 15** and add the IHC buffer containing primary antibodies at appropriate concentration. Incubate at least 4 h (*see* **Note 11**).

18. Remove the staining solution as described in **step 15**.

19. Transfer the slides to staining jars containing 50 ml of Tris buffer. Wash under gentle agitation for 5 min.

20. Remove the slides from the jar and absorb any excess of Tris buffer as described above (**step 15**).

21. Add 100–200 µl of IHC buffer containing secondary antibodies and incubate for at least 4 h.

22. Remove the staining solution (**step 15**), wash (**step 19**) and absorb any remaining buffer (**step 20**) as described above.

23. Mount the samples using an appropriate mounting medium (*see* **Note 12**).

3.2 Vibratome Sectioning

1. Follow **steps 1–5** of the protocol applicable for cryostat sectioning (Subheading 3.1).

2. Bring an aliquot of 4% agarose solution to 98 °C in a thermoshaker. Allow the solution to cool down until approximately 50 °C. Fill the histology mold with the liquid agarose solution. Avoid bubbles.

3. Embed the LN in the histology mold while the agarose is still liquid (*see* **Note 4**).

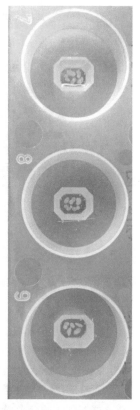

Fig. 1 Embedded LN (*see* **Notes 1** and **4–6**). Representative example of a histology mold carrier containing LN embedded in TFM

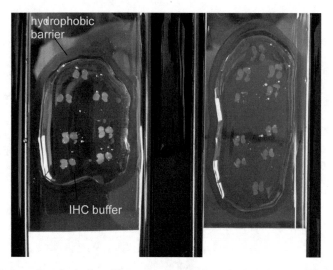

Fig. 2 Sample rehydration. Tissue sections were rehydrated using Tris buffer, which also removes TFM (*see* **Notes 9** and **10**)

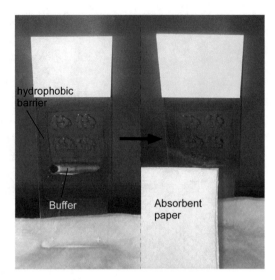

Fig. 3 Remove the remaining buffer in the hydrophobic pen area using gravity flow and paper tissue

4. Store the samples/embedded organs at 4 °C for 15 min to allow agarose polymerization.

5. Carefully remove the agarose-embedded sample from the histology mold using a scalpel blade (Fig. 4).

6. Fix the agarose block on the vibratome carrier using regular super glue (*see* **Note 13**).

7. Cut 200 μm thick sections using a vibratome set to an amplitude of 1.5 mm and a speed of 0.6 mm/s.

8. Place individual slices in 24 well plates containing 500 μl of Tris buffer (Fig. 5).

9. Remove the Tris buffer using a 1000 μl pipette.

10. Add 300 μl of IHC buffer per well. Incubate for 20 min with gentle agitation.

11. Remove the IHC buffer (*see* **step 9**) and add 300 μl of IHC buffer containing primary antibodies. Incubate at least 12 h (*see* **Note 11**).

12. Remove the staining solution as described above (**step 9**). Wash twice with 1 ml of Tris buffer.

13. Incubate with the IHC buffer containing secondary antibodies for at least 12 h (*see* **Note 14**).

14. Remove the staining solution and wash twice with 1 ml of Tris buffer.

15. Optional: Clarify the samples by adding 200–300 μl of Rapiclear 1.47® per slice. Incubate for 12 h minimum.

16. Mount slices in an appropriate mounting medium (*see* **Note 12**). If the tissue has been clarified (**step 15**), mount the slice in fresh Rapiclear 1.47®.

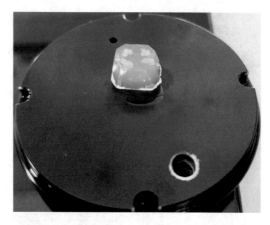

Fig. 4 Release of agarose-embedded sample block. A scalpel blade was put in position to carefully dissect the outer edges of the sample block (*see* **Note 13**)

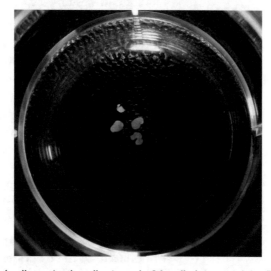

Fig. 5 Single slice cut using vibratome in 24 well plate containing Tris buffer

4   Notes

1. For optimal results, it is critical that adjacent tissues (fat, lymphatics, connective tissue) are carefully removed under a dissecting microscope before embedding.

2. Longer fixation should be avoided as it alters the binding of most antibodies.

3. During dehydration, make sure that LN do not stick to the tube or the cap. Sucrose is very sticky. Dehydration is complete when LN have sunk to the bottom of the tube, which usually takes a few hours.

4. While embedding in TFM (Subheading 3.1) and agarose (Subheading 3.2), avoid bubble formation. Any bubbles that might have formed should be carefully removed using a 200 µl pipette.

5. When multiple LN are embedded with TFM (Subheading 3.1) or agarose (Subheading 3.2) in the same histology mold, it is critical that they are (1) all at the bottom of the mold and (2) centered within the mold.

6. Embed a maximum of three inflamed or four non-inflamed LN per mold.

7. Freeze at least for 10 min. To accelerate the freezing process, place the molds in direct contact with the frozen steel of the freezer. Use of nitrogen is not necessary.

8. To remove TFM-embedded sample blocks from histology molds, hold the bottom of the mold between your fingertips. TFM will melt at the edge and removal will be easier.

9. In our experience, other slides yield suboptimal results. As they provide less adherence, sections tend to detach during the staining and washing steps.

10. Buffer should be added very carefully and slowly.

11. Dilution and incubation time need to be optimized for each organ and antibody. However, the conditions described here work for the detection of various antigens and thus, serve as a general guideline.

12. The choice of the mounting medium primarily depends on the fluorochromes conjugated to the antibodies used to stain the sections. Some mounting mediums alter the signal of specific fluorochromes.

13. For optimal sectioning results, ensure that the tissue block is placed on the vibratome carrier in a way that the cutting plane is even.

14. As for primary antibody staining, conditions for secondary antibodies need to be optimized for the specific reagents used. Generally, incubation with IHC buffer containing secondary antibodies for at least 12 h yields reliable results in our hands.

Acknowledgements

We would like to thank Delphine Suerinck for technical help. This work was supported by a grant from the European Research Council (ERC) under the European Union's Horizon 2020 research and innovation program grant agreement N° 647384-STROMA. The authors declare no conflict of interest.

References

1. Mueller SN, Germain RN (2009) Stromal cell contributions to the homeostasis and functionality of the immune system. Nat Rev Immunol 9(9):618–629. https://doi.org/10.1038/nri2588

2. Katakai T, Hara T, Sugai M, Gonda H, Shimizu A (2004) Lymph node fibroblastic reticular cells construct the stromal reticulum via contact with lymphocytes. J Exp Med 200(6):783–795

3. Kumar V, Chyou S, Stein JV, Lu TT (2012) Optical projection tomography reveals dynamics of HEV growth after immunization with protein plus CFA and features shared with HEVs in acute autoinflammatory lymphadenopathy. Front Immunol 3:282. https://doi.org/10.3389/fimmu.2012.00282

4. Chung K, Wallace J, Kim SY, Kalyanasundaram S, Andalman AS, Davidson TJ, Mirzabekov JJ, Zalocusky KA, Mattis J, Denisin AK, Pak S, Bernstein H, Ramakrishnan C, Grosenick L, Gradinaru V, Deisseroth K (2013) Structural and molecular interrogation of intact biological systems. Nature 497(7449):332–337. https://doi.org/10.1038/nature12107

5. Dodt HU, Leischner U, Schierloh A, Jahrling N, Mauch CP, Deininger K, Deussing JM, Eder M, Zieglgansberger W, Becker K (2007) Ultramicroscopy: three-dimensional visualization of neuronal networks in the whole mouse brain. Nat Methods 4(4):331–336. https://doi.org/10.1038/nmeth1036

6. Erturk A, Becker K, Jahrling N, Mauch CP, Hojer CD, Egen JG, Hellal F, Bradke F, Sheng M, Dodt HU (2012) Three-dimensional imaging of solvent-cleared organs using 3DISCO. Nat Protoc 7(11):1983–1995. https://doi.org/10.1038/nprot.2012.119

7. Hama H, Kurokawa H, Kawano H, Ando R, Shimogori T, Noda H, Fukami K, Sakaue-Sawano A, Miyawaki A (2011) Scale: a chemical approach for fluorescence imaging and reconstruction of transparent mouse brain. Nat Neurosci 14(11):1481–1488. https://doi.org/10.1038/nn.2928

8. Susaki EA, Tainaka K, Perrin D, Kishino F, Tawara T, Watanabe TM, Yokoyama C, Onoe H, Eguchi M, Yamaguchi S, Abe T, Kiyonari H, Shimizu Y, Miyawaki A, Yokota H, Ueda HR (2014) Whole-brain imaging with single-cell resolution using chemical cocktails and computational analysis. Cell 157(3):726–739. https://doi.org/10.1016/j.cell.2014.03.042

Chapter 7

Intravital Imaging of B Cell Responses in Lymph Nodes

Stefano Sammicheli, Mirela Kuka, and Matteo Iannacone

Abstract

Humoral immune responses depend on B cells encountering antigen (Ag) in lymph nodes (LNs) draining infection sites, getting activated, interacting with different cells, proliferating and differentiating into anti-body (Ab)-secreting cells. Each of these events occurs in distinct LN sub-compartments, requiring the migration of B cells from niche to niche in a fast and tightly coordinated fashion. While some of the rules that characterize B cell behavior in secondary lymphoid organs have been elucidated at the population level, we have only limited knowledge of the precise dynamics of B cell interactions with different kinds of LN cells at the single-cell level. Here, we describe in detail an intravital microscopy technique that allows the analysis of B cell dynamic behavior in the popliteal lymph node of anesthetized mice at high spatial and temporal resolution. A detailed understanding of the spatiotemporal dynamics of B cells within secondary lymphoid organs may lead to novel, rational vaccine strategies aimed at inducing rapid and long-lived humoral immune responses.

Key words Multiphoton intravital microscopy, In vivo imaging, Lymph Node, B cells, Antibody, Antiviral immunity, Lymphocyte motility

1 Introduction

Antibody responses rely on B cells encountering Ag, interacting with helper T cells and dendritic cells, proliferating and differentiating into high-affinity plasma cells and memory B cells. Each of these actions take place in distinct niches of secondary lymphoid organs, necessitating the migration of B cells among different sub-compartments in a rapid and extremely coordinated manner [1]. Early understanding of the initiation of humoral immune responses in LNs has been based on static imaging techniques such as immunohistochemistry and electron microscopy [2–4]. In recent years, the advent of multiphoton intravital microscopy (MP-IVM) has taken the field to a whole new level, enabling the dynamic visualization of B cells within secondary lymphoid tissue in vivo [5, 6]. Through the use of MP-IVM several ground-breaking studies have

Masaru Ishii (ed.), *Intravital Imaging of Dynamic Bone and Immune Systems: Methods and Protocols*, Methods in Molecular Biology, vol. 1763, https://doi.org/10.1007/978-1-4939-7762-8_7, © Springer Science+Business Media, LLC 2018

started to shed new light on the way by which B cells encounter Ag and become activated in LNs (reviewed in [5, 7–10]).

Here, we detail an intravital microscopy method to study B cell dynamics within the popliteal lymph node (popLN) at the single-cell level. The protocol begins with a description of lymphocyte isolation, purification, labeling with fluorescent dyes and subsequent intravenous injection into recipient mice. It then provides a step-by-step surgical procedure to expose the popLN for intravital microscopy using an upright microscope setup (originally developed by the von Andrian laboratory [11]), accompanied by protocols validated by our group to image motility and functions of lymphocytes in popLN. Finally, it describes the basic analyses of intravital microscopy movies to compute several motility parameters.

2   Materials

2.1   Preparation and Injection of Control Wild Type (WT) and BCR Transgenic (tg) B Cells, as Well as CD4+ T Cells to be Tracked In Vivo

- Spleens and LNs from donor WT or BCR tg mice. Donors should be from the same genetic background as the recipients (e.g., C57BL/6).
- Sterile cell strainer, size: 70 μm.
- Ammonium-Chloride-Potassium (ACK) lysis buffer (prepared in house).
- Hank's balanced salt solution (HBSS).
- Roswell Park Memorial Institute (RPMI) 1640.
- Immunomagnetic cell purification kit for naïve B cells (e.g., mouse CD43⁻ untouched naïve B cell negative selection kit).
- Immunomagnetic cell purification kit for naïve CD4+ T cells (e.g., mouse CD4+ T cell isolation kit).
- Miltenyi Biotec separation buffer (prepared according to the manufacturer's instructions).
- Cell tracker dyes: 5-chloromethylfluorescein diacetate (CMFDA, CellTracker™ Green), CellTracker™ Red (CMTPX), 5-(and-6)-(((4-chloromethyl) benzoyl) amino) tetramethylrhodamine (CMTMR, CellTracker™ Orange), CellTracker™ Deep Red, 6-(((4,4-difluoro-5-(2-thienyl)-4-bora-3a,4a–diaza-s-indacene-3-yl)styryloxy)acetyl) aminohexanoic acid (BODIPY 630/650-X).
- Mouse restrainer.

2.2   Surgical Anesthesia

- Isoflurane (*see* **Note 1**).
- Anesthetic vaporizers (I) (Fig. 1a).
- Acepromazine maleate.

A

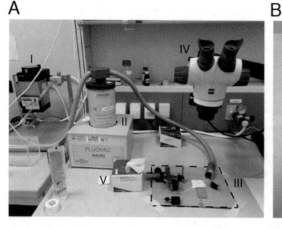

B

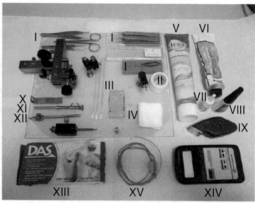

Fig. 1 *Equipment required for the popliteal LN surgery.* (**a**) Surgical area equipped with oxygen supply connected to the isoflurane vaporizer (I), isoflurane trap (II), surgical stage (III), stereomicroscope (IV), and precision wipes (V). (**b**) Surgical equipment: surgical instruments (I), medical adhesive tape (II), cotton-tipped applicators (III), gauze sponges (IV), hair removal cream (V), high-viscosity vacuum grease (VI), tissue glue (VII), ethyl-2-cyanoacrylate glue (VIII), small-animal clipper (IX), coverslip support (X), spine-holding clamp (XI), upper leg bone-holding clamp (XII), plasticine modeling clay (XIII), digital thermometer (XIV), and miniature K type thermocouples (XV)

- Oxygen supply connected to the isoflurane vaporizer.
- Isoflurane Trap (II) (Fig. 1a) (Fluovac 240 VAC, 50 Hz).

2.3 Surgical Preparation of the Mouse Popliteal Lymph Node for Intravital Microscopy Using an Upright Microscope Setup

- Custom-built stag.5e (III) (described in [12]).
- Stereomicroscope (IV) (e.g., Zeiss CL 1500 Eco, from Zeiss) (Fig. 1a).
- Surgical instruments (I) (e.g., from Fine Science Tools, Foster City, CA, USA): Spring scissors (Cohan-Vannas 6 mm blade); Extra thin iris scissors (10.5 cm); Dumont #2 laminectomy forceps Inox; Adson forceps (12 cm); Standard pattern scissors (large loops, sharp/blunt 14.5 cm); Extra thin tweezers (Dumont #5SF Forceps) (Fig. 1b).
- Medical adhesive tape (II) (Fig. 1b).
- 15 cm cotton-tipped applicators (III) (Fig. 1b).
- Gauze sponges (IV) (Fig. 1b).
- Hair removal cream (V) (Fig. 1b).
- High-viscosity vacuum grease (VI) (Fig. 1b).
- Tissue glue (VII) (Fig. 1b).
- Ethyl-2-cyanoacrylate glue (VIII) (Fig. 1b).
- Small-animal clipper (IX) (Fig. 1b).
- Precision Wipes (V) (11 × 21 cm) (Fig. 1a).
- Suture thread: 5-0 braided silk (suture size), C-1 (needle type), 13.1 mm (needle length), 3/8c (needle shape).

- Coverslip support (X), spine-holding clamp (XI) and upper leg bone-holding clamp (XII) (Fig. 1b).
- Round glass coverslips (24 mm in diameter, 0.17 mm thickness).
- Plasticine modeling clay (XIII) (Fig. 1b).
- Digital thermometer (XIV) and miniature K type thermocouples (XV) (Fig. 1b).

2.4 Multiphoton Intravital Microscopy of the Mouse Popliteal Lymph Node Using an Upright Microscope Setup

- Upright multiphoton microscope equipped with: (a) at least one (preferably two) tunable femtosecond (fs)-pulsed Ti:Sa lasers (e.g., 680–1080 nm, 120 fs pulse-width, 80 MHz repetition rate, Ultra II, Coherent, Santa Clara, CA, USA); (b) an optional Optical Parametric Oscillator (e.g., 1000–1600 nm, 200 fs pulse-width, 80 MHz repetition rate, Chameleon Compact OPO, Coherent, Santa Clara, CA); (c) at least two (ideally four or five) non-descanned photomultiplier tubes (e.g., Hamamatsu H7422-40 GaAsP High Sensitivity PMTs and Hamamatsu H7422-50 GaAsP High Sensitivity red-extended PMT from Hamamatsu Photonics K.K., Hamamatsu city, Japan); (d) a high numerical aperture, water-immersion multiphoton objective (preferably Olympus ref.: XLPLN25XWMP2, 25×, 1.05 NA, 2 mm working distance, Center Valley PA, USA).
- Mercury arc lamp (e.g., X-cite 120Q-Wide-Field Fluorescence Microscope Light Source, from Excelitas, New York City, USA).
- Custom-made thermostatic chamber that surrounds the entire microscope with the exclusion of the scanhead.
- Digital thermometer (XIV) (Fig. 1b).

2.5 Image Acquisition, Processing, and Analysis

- Computer workstation with high graphics processing capability (e.g., Apple Inc. (Cupertino, CA, USA) Computer model: Mac Pro: Processor: 2 × 2.4 GHz Quad-core Intel Xeon or higher, Memory: 32 GB 1066 MHz DDR3 ECC, Graphics: ATI Radeon HD 5870 1024 MB, System: MAC OS X Lion 10.7 or higher).
- Image analysis software (e.g., Imaris, Bitplane, Zurich, Switzerland; Volocity, Improvision, Coventry, UK; ImageJ, National Institute of Health, Bethesda, MD) and eventual custom-made scripts (Matlab, Mathworks, Natick, MA, USA or Python, Beaverton, OR, USA) for more complicated analyses.

3   Methods

3.1 Preparation and Injection of B Cells to be Tracked In Vivo

- Spleens and LNs are gently dissociated in HBSS, filtered through a 70 μm cell strainer and red blood cells are lysed by using the ACK lysis buffer to obtain a single cell suspension.

- Untouched naïve CD43$^-$ B cells or CD4$^+$ T cells from single cell suspensions of LNs and spleens are purified by negative immunomagnetic selection, according to the manufacturer's instructions.

- Naïve B cells and CD4$^+$ T cells are washed on pre-warmed serum-free RPMI to remove residual FBS. Cells are incubated at 1×10^7 cells/ml and stained with 2.5 μM CMFDA, 7.5 μM CMTPX, 10 μM CMTMR, CellTracker™ Deep Red, or 2.5 μM BODIPY 630/650-X for 20 min in the dark at 37 °C in plain pre-warmed RPMI 1640. The reaction is stopped with addition of 2 ml of FBS, which binds residual protein-binding dyes. The cells are then washed twice with pre-warmed RPMI and resuspended in PBS at the desired concentration (typically between 10^7 and 10^8 cells/ml). As an alternative to cell staining with fluorescent organic dyes, B cells and CD4$^+$ T cells can be isolated from mice expressing a fluorescent protein (e.g., green fluorescent protein or its variants) under a ubiquitous or cell-specific promoter.

- Fluorescently labeled naïve B cells and CD4$^+$ T cells are injected intravenously into recipient mice through the tail vein (typically between 5×10^6 and 2×10^7 of each cell population per mouse) and allowed to home to secondary lymphoid organs for ~18 h.

3.2 Microscope Setup and Presurgical Preparations

- Turn the system on (set the thermal chamber at 37 °C, turn on the computer, lasers, mercury arc lamp, open the oxygen supply connected to the isoflurane vaporizer system, and check the isoflurane volume).

- Stage preparation. Fix the stage to the bench at the four corners with medical adhesive tape (Fig. 1a). Place a gauze sponge in the middle of the stage where the mouse will be rested (Fig. 1a).

- The right mouse leg, flank, and the back are shaved using clippers and depilation crème is applied briefly (<30 s) to the right leg, avoiding skin irritation. Thoroughly wipe off the crème using moist gauze and repeat if required. The goal is to remove hairs entirely as they are very autofluorescent and therefore can interfere with imaging (see **Note 1**).

3.3 Surgical Anesthesia

The mouse is injected with 10 μg of Acepromazine maleate ~45 min prior to the surgical procedure (see **Note 2**). The mouse is then anesthetized with 5% isoflurane through a nose cone also delivering oxygen at 1 L/min (see **Note 3**). Adequate anesthesia is achieved if the mouse does not react to firm pinching of the footpad. Follow-up surgery and popLN intravital imaging are carried out with lower concentrations of isoflurane (between 0.8% and 1%). Anesthesia is adjusted based on breathing rate (~55–65 breaths per minute).

3.4 Surgical Preparation for popLN Intravital Microscopy
(See Note 4)

- Place the mouse on the microscope stage and secure the anesthesia nose cone by using adhesive tape. Then position the mouse on the stage using adhesive tape attached to the left hind leg, the left fore leg, and the tip of the tail (Fig. 2a).

- Pull the mouse leg by using a sling of suture thread attached to one of the toes (Fig. 2b).

- Pull the tail with the tape over the back of the mouse and identify the tip of the right greater trochanter (a prominent bony pivot of the upper leg bone) through palpation and gently perform a midline 1 cm skin incision in the flank (Fig. 2c).

- Cut the attached connective tissue and apply the first holding clamp. During this, the right leg should be in a rotational position so that the popliteal fat pad, which is visible through the skin, is facing straight upward (Fig. 2d).

- Close the incision by applying tissue glue on the skin surrounding the holding clamp.

- The dorsal skin is incised over a distance of about 1 cm to expose the upper lumbar spine (Fig. 2e) and a small fraction of its circumference freed of the attached musculature. The second holding clamp is attached to the spine's dorsal aspect (Fig. 2f).

- Close the incision by applying tissue glue on the skin surrounding the holding clamp. Now the mouse is well stabilized and the microsurgery to expose the popLN can begin (Fig. 2g).

- Using the iris scissors and with the help of a stereomicroscope, the skin overlying the popLN is longitudinally incised over a length of about 1 cm, using the popliteal vein as a landmark structure (Fig. 2h). From this moment onwards, the surgical area should be kept moist by creating a little pool with high-viscosity vacuum grease and applying small amounts of saline solution (NaCl 0.9%) (see Note 5).

- Through blunt dissection, using the fine forceps, gently tease away some of the connective and fat tissue to the left of the lateral marginal vein so that the popLN is readily exposed (Fig. 2i–k).

Fig. 2 (continued) (**g**) Overview of the mouse on the surgical stage. (**h**) Longitudinal incision of the skin overlaying the popliteal LN and exposure of the popliteal vein. (**i**) Plasticine blocks molded onto both side of the leg create a gentle pressure onto the mouse leg helping the exposure of the popliteal LN (arrow and dashed line). The popliteal LN is constantly submerged in saline solution via a little pool created with high-viscosity vacuum grease. (**j**) Final exposure position of the popliteal LN (arrow and dashed line). (**k**) Evans blue injected subcutaneously into the footpad highlights the afferent lymphatic vessel (arrow). The popliteal LN is denoted by a dashed line. (**l**) Coverslip (dashed line) glued to the micropositioning device creates a closed chamber with the pool of saline solution and is gently lowered until in contact with the upper surface of the exposed popliteal LN at the center of the coverslip (arrow and dashed line). (**m**) Overview of the mouse preparation and positioning of the thermocouple probe (arrow) prior to imaging acquisition

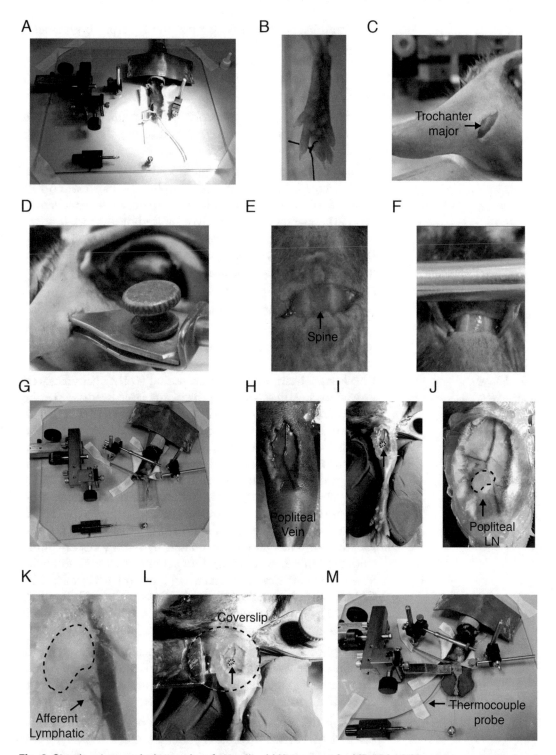

Fig. 2 *Step-by-step surgical procedure for popliteal LN exposure for MP-IVM.* (**a**) Mouse is anesthetized and positioned on its right flank. (**b**) Suture thread is attached to the toe. (**c**) Skin incision on the flank and exposure of the right trochanter major. (**d**) Positioning of the holding clamp on the right trochanter major. (**e**) Dorsal skin incision and exposure of the upper lumbar spine. (**f**) Positioning of the holding clamp on the spine.

- Plasticine blocks are molded onto the leg from both sides at the level of the popLN. Applying gentle pressure from both sides pushes the popLN into a slightly elevated position that makes it more accessible during tissue dissection (Fig. 2i–k) (*see* **Note 6**).

- Lubricate the temperature probe with vacuum grease prior to inserting into the mouse rectum and secure the probe to the stage with adhesive tape.

- A clean coverslip glued to a micropositioning device mounted on the stage is lowered onto the popliteal fossa to seal off the pool of saline solution and thus create a closed chamber (Fig. 2l). Take special care to avoid air bubbles as they interfere with imaging. The coverglass can gently touch the upper surface of the popLN, but excessive pressure should be avoided as it might impair blood perfusion.

- Create a second ring of high-viscosity vacuum grease along the perimeter of the coverslip and apply distilled water.

- Transfer the stage to the intravital microscope into the 37 °C pre-warmed thermal chamber (Fig. 2m).

3.5 Image Acquisition

- Check laser beam alignment according to the manufacturer's instructions. Adjust wavelengths of the laser beams according to the fluorescent dyes used in the experiment (two photon excitation spectra of most commonly used fluorescent probes can be found, e.g., at http://goo.gl/4qYhWx). Typically, we tune the two Ti:Sa lasers at 800 nm and 900–930 nm, respectively, and the OPO at 1200 nm. This setup allows us to excite most fluorescent molecules whose emission range from ~450 nm to ~700 nm. Spectral separation is achieved by dichromatic mirrors and bandpass filters in front of each PMTs. Again, selection of filters should be guided by the fluorescent molecules used in the experiment. Our setup includes the following filters: 455/50 nm (to detect, e.g., second harmonic, CFP, CMAC, Hoechst), 525/50 nm (to detect, e.g., eGFP, CFSE, CMFDA), 590/50 nm (to detect, e.g., CMTMR, dsRed) and 665/50 nm (to detect, e.g., BODIPY, qDots 655).

- As lymphocyte migration is highly temperature dependent, the thermostatic chamber is kept at 37–38 °C and the mouse body temperature is continuously monitored through a rectal probe to ensure that a narrow range of 37–38 °C is maintained at all time.

- Through the microscope eyepieces the popLN can be distinguished from the surrounding tissue structures by its ovoid shape and its green autofluorescence under mercury arc lamp illumination. The robustness of perfusion can also be assessed by visualizing negatively contrasted blood vessels.

- Before beginning image acquisition, several parameters (including laser power, PMT gain, offset, etc.) have to be adjusted in order to get the best possible signal-to-noise ratio. Acquisition of a test short time-lapse recording is advised, in order to check stability of the preparation (with particular attention to z-drift) and proper cell motility.

- The second harmonic signal originating from the collagen (blue fibers in Fig. 3a) delineates the LN capsule and serves as a convenient anatomical landmark for orientation in the tissue. Naïve B cells at steady state localize underneath the capsule in B cell follicles (Fig. 3a, inset 1) whereas CD4+ T cells reside in the T cell area deeper into the LN parenchyma (Fig. 3a, inset 2).

- Once an area of interest is found, actual recording can begin. Typically, we found that stacks of ~10–11 square xy sections (512×512 pixels) sampled with ~4 µm z spacing acquired every ~10 s for a period of ~30–40 min provide a sufficient amount of cell tracks for meaningful statistical analyses. Our experimental setup allows for continuous recording for at least 4–5 h.

3.6 Image Processing and Analysis

Initially, the sequences of image stacks are transformed into volume-rendered 4D time-lapse movies with image analysis software (e.g., Imaris Bitplane or Fiji ImageJ). The 3D positions of the cell centroids are segmented by semiautomated cell tracking algorithm from Imaris or using the TrackMate Fiji plugin. Typically, the data can provide qualitative and quantitative information on cell localization, track analyses, and interactive behavior relative to other cell types.

1. Track analysis. Several different motility parameters can be quantified, including:

   - Instant velocity (Fig. 3b): Velocity of B cells or CD4+ T cells calculated as displacement/time during a single time step.

   - Mean velocity (Fig. 3c): mean velocity of a cell over several time steps (usually the entire imaging period, in µm/min).

   - Track length (Fig. 3d): Cumulative distance (distance [d] 1 + d2 + d3, etc.) traveled by a cell over a given time (in µm).

   - Displacement (Fig. 3d): Distance between the first and the last imaging point (in µm).

   - Meandering index (Fig. 3e): The ratio between the displacement and the total track length. It is a measure of the straightness (or confinement) of cell tracks. It can vary between 0 (if the cell returns to the exact position where it started) and 1 (in case of a perfectly straight cell track).

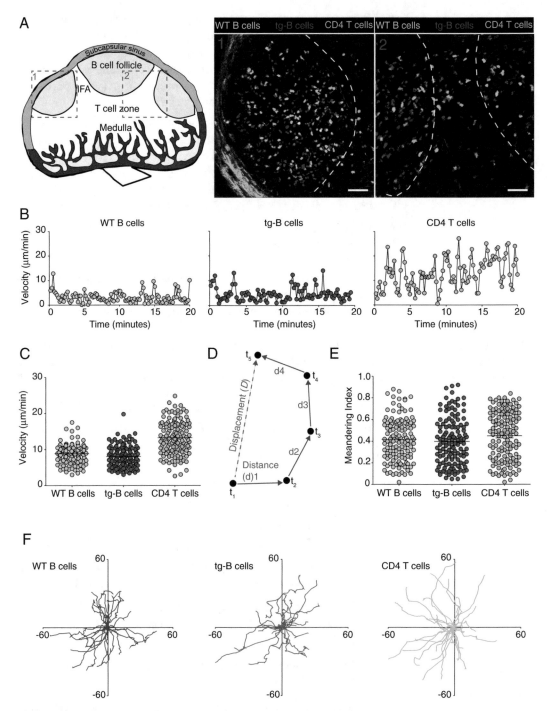

Fig. 3 *MP-IVM data analyses.* (**a**) (Left panel) Schematic representation of a cross-sectional view of the popliteal LN highlighting the subcapsular sinus, B cell follicles, interfollicular areas (IFA), T cell zone, and medulla. (Middle and right panels) Multiphoton intravital micrographs in the popliteal LN of a WT mouse that was injected with WT (cyan) and transgenic (red) B cells as well as with CD4⁺ T cells (green) 18 h prior to imaging acquisition. Micrographs are snapshots by MP-IVM of two areas of the popLN (1 and 2) denoted by the dashed red quadrant in left panel. Dotted white line denotes B cell follicles. Scale bars represent 50 μm (middle and right panels).

2. Migratory behavior and directionality. Cell populations can be qualitatively examined by plotting the trajectories of the tracked cell centroids over time in two dimensions. The first position of each individual cell is shifted to the same starting point in space (Fig. 3f) while maintaining its orientation, allowing to assess whether cells are traveling in a preferred direction. If all possible directions are equally covered, this indicates that motion is random on the timescale of the duration of the plotted tracks (plotting tracks only give qualitative information).

4   Notes

1. As mouse shaving requires the use of isoflurane, we usually perform it a day before the imaging session (in order to limit isoflurane exposure right before the surgery). It is important to thoroughly rinse off the hair removal cream and hair fragments with PBS as they are autofluorescent and can interfere with imaging. Moreover, long exposure to hair removal cream can induce undesirable skin inflammation.

2. Acepromazine maleate is a sedative drug and a potent myorelaxant. Treatment of mice with low doses of Acepromazine helps in preventing muscle contractions that might cause motion artifacts.

3. Although injectable anesthetics can be used in place of inhalational anesthetics, we favor the latter ones because they can be adjusted quickly as needed during the experiment, they allow for longer imaging sessions and for more physiological heart rate, breathing rate, and hemodynamic parameters.

4. Although other skin-draining LNs have been used for intravital imaging, we favor the popliteal LN because it is the smallest skin-draining LN and because motion artifacts caused by respiratory movements can be more easily minimized.

5. The surgical procedure to expose the popLN will take ~30 min during which time the surgical area must always be submerged with saline solution at 37 °C. The saline solution must be

---

Fig. 3 (continued) (**b**) Instantaneous velocity (μm/min [min]) of WT (cyan) and transgenic (red) B cells or CD4+ T cells (green) evaluated in a WT mouse injected as described in (**a**). (**b**) Mean velocity (μm/min) of WT (cyan) and transgenic (red) B cells or CD4+ T cells (green) evaluated in a WT mouse injected as described in (**a**). (**c**) Schematic showing the distance of a cell (d_1, d_2, etc.) at five consecutive time points (t_1, t_2, etc.). The displacement (D) of a cell is the shortest distance between the positions at two time points (which is distinct from the length of the entire path it has traveled). (**d**) Meandering index of WT (cyan) and transgenic (red) B cells or CD4+ T cells (green) evaluated in a WT mouse injected as described in (**a**). (**e**) The same mouse described in (**a**) was subjected to MP-IVM in the popliteal LN. Track plots of individual WT (cyan) and transgenic (red) B cells or CD4+ T cells (green) were recorded during a 45-min observation period. Each track has been shifted such that it starts at the origin of the x and y axes

changed regularly as it gets easily muddled by the tissue damage required by the surgery.

6. The microsurgical procedure can be a technical challenge and it might require some training to master. Special care should be taken to prevent afferent lymph vessel disruption. This can be learned by performing several training surgeries upon footpad injection of a dye (e.g., Evans blue) to outline the lymphatic vasculature (Fig. 2k). Typically, at least three afferent lymph vessels can be identified entering the popLN during the procedure. Blunt dissection (insertion of closed forceps or scissors into the tissue followed by their opening) minimizes bleeding. A certain degree of bleeding from superficial blood vessels may occur during the procedure and it is tolerated as it will not affect popLN perfusion (which occurs through deeper arteries). Superficial bleeding can usually be stopped by grabbing and applying pressure on the vessel with forceps for ~30 s.

References

1. Pereira JP, Kelly LM, Cyster JG (2010) Finding the right niche: B-cell migration in the early phases of T-dependent antibody responses. Int Immunol 22:413–419. https://doi.org/10.1093/intimm/dxq047

2. Andrian v UH, Mempel TR (2003) Homing and cellular traffic in lymph nodes. Nat Rev Immunol 3:867–878. https://doi.org/10.1038/nri1222

3. Halin C, Mora JR, Sumen C, Andrian v UH (2005) In vivo imaging of lymphocyte trafficking. Annu Rev Cell Dev Biol 21:581–603. https://doi.org/10.1146/annurev.cellbio.21.122303.133159

4. Bajénoff M, Egen JG, Qi H et al (2007) Highways, byways and breadcrumbs: directing lymphocyte traffic in the lymph node. Trends Immunol 28:346–352. https://doi.org/10.1016/j.it.2007.06.005

5. Batista FD, Harwood NE (2009) The who, how and where of antigen presentation to B cells. Nat Rev Immunol 9:15–27. https://doi.org/10.1038/nri2454

6. Germain RN, Robey EA, Cahalan MD (2012) A decade of imaging cellular motility and interaction dynamics in the immune system. Science 336:1676–1681. https://doi.org/10.1126/science.1221063

7. Cyster JG (2010) B cell follicles and antigen encounters of the third kind. Nat Immunol 11:989–996. https://doi.org/10.1038/ni.1946

8. Kuka M, Iannacone M (2014) The role of lymph node sinus macrophages in host defense. Ann N Y Acad Sci 1319:38–46. https://doi.org/10.1111/nyas.12387

9. Gonzalez SF, Degn SE, Pitcher LA et al (2011) Trafficking of B cell antigen in lymph nodes. Annu Rev Immunol 29:215–233. https://doi.org/10.1146/annurev-immunol-031210-101255

10. Victora GD, Mesin L (2014) Clonal and cellular dynamics in germinal centers. Curr Opin Immunol 28C:90–96. https://doi.org/10.1016/j.coi.2014.02.010

11. Mempel TR, Henrickson SE, Andrian v UH (2004) T-cell priming by dendritic cells in lymph nodes occurs in three distinct phases. Nature 427:154–159. https://doi.org/10.1038/nature02238

12. Murooka TT, Mempel TR (2012) Multiphoton intravital microscopy to study lymphocyte motility in lymph nodes. Methods Mol Biol 757:247–257. https://doi.org/10.1007/978-1-61779-166-6_16

Chapter 8

Live Imaging of the Skin Immune Responses: Visualization of the Contact Hypersensitivity Response

Gyohei Egawa, Tetsuya Honda, and Kenji Kabashima

Abstract

A variety of immune cells are involved in cutaneous immune responses. Over the last decade, intravital imaging has become an important technique used to capture the dynamic behavior of immune cells in the physiological context. In this chapter, we describe essential techniques for visualizing immune cells in the skin, focusing on the contact hypersensitivity response. Using fluorescent dyes and transgenic reporter animals, many kinds of immune cells and skin components can be visualized in three dimensions and in a noninvasive manner.

Key words Multiphoton microscopy, T cell, Dendritic cell, Contact hypersensitivity

1 Introduction

A variety of immune cells, including T cells, granulocytes, dendritic cells, and macrophages, move actively throughout the body to scan for pathogens. To capture this dynamic immune cell behavior, intravital imaging has become an essential technique. Multiphoton (MP) microscopy (also referred to as two-photon excitation microscopy) was first demonstrated by Denk et al. [1] and has been used in the field of immunology since the mid-2000s. Compared with conventional single-photon excitation microscopes, MP microscopes allow deeper tissue penetration with less photodamage, achieving high spatio-temporal resolution. These features made MP microscopes as standard devices for the intravital imaging of biological specimens.

The skin covers the entire body and protects us from the external environment. Many kinds of cutaneous immune responses have been visualized by intravital imaging [2]. Transgenic animals that express fluorescent reporter protein in specific cells have been used to visualize skin-resident cells, such as Langerhans cells (Langerin-eGFP mice), dendritic cells (CD11c-eYFP mice), neutrophils/macrophages (LysM-eGFP mice), and γδT cells (CXCR6-eGFP

Masaru Ishii (ed.), *Intravital Imaging of Dynamic Bone and Immune Systems: Methods and Protocols*, Methods in Molecular Biology, vol. 1763, https://doi.org/10.1007/978-1-4939-7762-8_8, © Springer Science+Business Media, LLC 2018

Table 1
Transgenic mice available for intravital imaging of the skin

Promoter	Reporter	Type	Target cell	Reference
Ubiquitous				
CAG/chicken β actin	EGFP	Tg	Ubiquitous	[7]
CAG	Kaede/KikGR	Tg	Ubiquitous (photoconvertible)	[8, 9]
Bone marrow-derived				
CD11c	EYFP	Tg	DC	[10]
Langerin	EGFP	KI	Langerhans cell, Langerin+ dermal DC	[11]
Lysozyme M	EGFP	KI	Neutrophil, monocyte, macrophage	[10, 12]
DPE	GFP	Tg	Macrophage, pDC, T cell	[12]
CSF-1R	EGFP	Tg	Neutrophil, monocyte, macrophage	[10]
IL-1β	DsRed	Tg	Langerhans cell	[13]
Mcpt5	YFP	Cre/loxp	Mast cell	[14]
TCRδ/CXCR6	EGFP	KI	γδ T cell	[15, 16]
Others				
Tie2	GFP	Tg	Blood vessel	[17]
Prox1	EGFP	Tg	Lymphatic vessel	[18]
Thy1.2	EGFP	Tg	Neuron	[19]

mice) (Table 1). To visualize skin-infiltrating αβT cells, the adoptive transfer of labeled αβT cells is the standard technique because very few αβT cells are resident in the skin and αβT cells need to be activated to infiltrate the skin.

In this chapter, we describe (1) an essential procedure for cutaneous immune imaging and (2) how to visualize skin-infiltrating T cells in the context of the contact hypersensitivity (CHS) response. The CHS response, a prototypic T cell-mediated delayed-type (type IV) hypersensitivity response, is one of the most extensively studied immune responses in the skin [3, 4]. A schema of the CHS response is shown in Fig. 1. Lastly, we describe (3) how to visualize cutaneous blood vessels with fluorescent dye.

2   Materials

2.1   Method for Cutaneous Immune Imaging

1. Six- to eight-week-old mice (*see* **Notes 1–3**).

2. A two-photon microscope with a tunable (690–1040 nm) Ti/sapphire laser (Mai Tai DeepSee, Spectra-Physics, Santa Clara, CA, USA) (*see* **Note 4**).

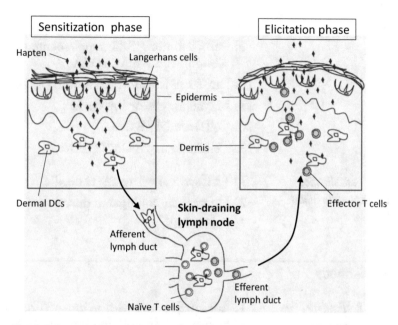

Fig. 1 Schematic representation of a CHS reaction. In the sensitization phase, hapten-bearing dendritic cells (DCs) migrate into draining lymph node and present antigens to naïve T cells. In the elicitation phase, activated-effector T cells infiltrate into the skin and interact with cutaneous DCs

3. Inhalation anesthesia apparatus for small animals.

4. Hair removal cream (*see* **Note 5**).

5. Pentobarbital sodium: 10% (v/v) solution in phosphate buffered saline (PBS) (*see* **Note 6**).

6. Cover glass (24 mm × 24 mm/24 mm × 50 mm).

7. Isoflurane.

8. Grease.

9. Immersion oil.

2.2 Intravital Imaging of Skin-Infiltrating T Cells

1. Standard equipment to collect lymph nodes, including cell culture dishes, a 40-μm nylon cell strainer, 1 ml syringe, 15 ml centrifuge tubes, and 1 ml microcentrifuge tubes.

2. Electric shaver.

3. 2,4-Dinitrofluorobenzene (DNFB) (*see* **Note 7**).

4. Olive oil.

5. Acetone.

6. 2% RPMI: RPMI 1640 medium supplemented with 2% fetal calf serum.

7. 10% RPMI: RPMI 1640 medium supplemented with 10% fetal calf serum Sterile PBS: 1.37 M NaCl, 0.027 M KCl, 0.081 M Na_2HPO_4, 0.0147 M KH_2PO_4.

8. PBS.

9. MACS buffer: PBS supplemented with 0.5% bovine serum albumin and 2 mM EDTA.

10. Pan T cell isolation kit, mouse (*see* **Note 8**).

11. Magnetic cell-sorting device.

12. CellTrace CFSE dye.

13. CellTracker Red CMTPX dye.

2.3 Visualization of Cutaneous Blood Vessels

1. 1 ml syringe with a 23 G needle.

2. Fluorescein-conjugated dextran (150 kDa).

3. Sterile PBS.

3 Methods

3.1 Method for Cutaneous Immune Imaging

3.1.1 Mouse Preparation

1. Anesthetize mice with an intraperitoneal injection of 10% pentobarbital sodium solution (10 μl per g body weight) (*see* **Note 9**).

2. Apply hair removal cream to the ventral and dorsal side of the left ear skin. Three minutes later, remove the cream from the ear using wet cotton or running water (*see* **Note 10**).

3. Apply the grease to the dorsal side of the left ear using a cotton swab (*see* **Note 11**).

4. Attach the 24 mm × 24 mm cover glass to the dorsal side of the left ear.

3.1.2 Placing the Mouse onto the Microscope Stage (Fig. 2)

Place the mouse on a heating pad at 37 °C throughout the imaging procedure.

1. If necessary, place a single drop of immersion oil on the objective lens.

2. Cover the central hole of the microscope stage with a 24 mm × 50 mm cover glass and fix it with tape (*see* **Note 12**).

3. Place a drop of immersion oil onto the cover glass immediately above the objective lens.

4. Place a mouse onto the stage. Sandwich the ear between two cover glasses (*see* **Note 13**).

5. Connect the mouse to the anesthetic apparatus. Flow 1% isoflurane at a rate of 1 L/min (*see* **Note 14**).

6. Stabilize the mouse using tape.

3.1.3 Start Imaging

1. Set the appropriate excitation laser wavelength. The ideal excitation wavelength is 940–960 nm for EYFP and EGFP and 780–800 nm for CFSE and CMTPX [5]. Collagen fibers in the dermis can be visualized by second harmonic generation.

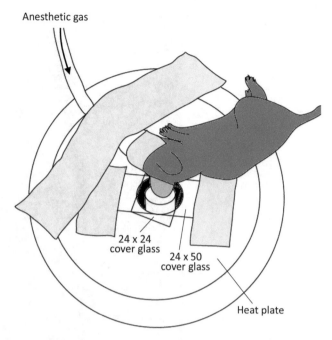

Anesthetic gas

24 x 24
cover glass

24 x 50
cover glass

Heat plate

Fig. 2 Fix mouse on the stage. The ear lobe is sandwiched between two cover slips. Mouse sensitization

2. Commence imaging. We typically take stacks of 15–20 images, spaced 3.5 μm apart, every 1–5 min for 3–12 h (*see* **Note 15**).

3.2 Intravital Imaging of Skin-Infiltrating T Cells

Before sensitizing mice, keep mice calm in a cage for at least 24 h (*see* **Note 16**).

3.2.1 Sensitize Mice with Hapten

1. Prepare 0.5% (w/v) DNFB solution (*see* **Notes 6** and **17**).

2. Shave the abdominal hair thoroughly using an electric shaver (*see* **Note 18**).

3. Hold the mouse in one hand and paint 25 μl of 0.5% DNFB solution on the shaved abdomen (Fig. 3) (*see* **Note 19**).

4. Air-dry the DNFB solution.

5. Sensitize at least five mice (*see* **Note 20**).

6. Keep the mice calm for 5 days (*see* **Note 21**).

3.2.2 Preparation of Single Cell Suspension of Lymph Node Cells

All buffers should be kept on ice (>10 °C).

1. Euthanize mice with the proper procedure.

2. Collect both sides of the axillary and inguinal lymph nodes (*see* **Note 22**). Put lymph nodes into 5 ml of 2% RPMI in a 15 ml centrifuge tube and keep on ice.

3. Using a syringe plunger, mash the lymph nodes through a 40-μm cell strainer.

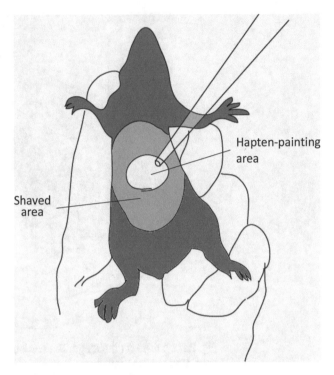

Hapten-painting area

Shaved area

Fig. 3 Hold a mouse in one hand and paint the hapten solution onto the shaved abdomen as shown

4. Centrifuge at 3000 × *g* for 3 min at 4 °C and discard supernatant.

5. Resuspend cells in 10 ml of MACS buffer.

6. Count cells (*see* **Note 23**).

7. Centrifuge at 3000 × *g* for 3 min at 4 °C and discard supernatant.

3.2.3   Isolation of T Cells with a Magnetic Cell Sorter

1. Resuspend cells in 40 μl of MACS buffer per 10^7 cells.

2. Add 10 μl of biotin-antibody cocktail per 10^7 cells.

3. Mix well and incubate for 5 min on ice.

4. Add 10 ml of MACS buffer.

5. Centrifuge at 3000 × *g* for 3 min at 4 °C and discard supernatant.

6. Resuspend cells in 80 μl of MACS buffer per 10^7 cells.

7. Add 20 μl of anti-biotin microbeads per 10^7 cells.

8. Mix well and incubate for 10 min on ice.

9. Wash cells as in **steps 4** and **5**.

10. Resuspend cells in 1 ml MACS buffer.

11. To remove cell clumps, filter the cell suspension through a 40-μm cell strainer.

12. Isolate T cells with a magnetic cell sorter (*see* **Note 24**).

13. Count cells (*see* **Note 25**).

14. Centrifuge at 3000 × *g* for 3 min at 4 °C and discard supernatant.

3.2.4 Cell Labeling with Fluorescent Dyes

1. Resuspend cells in 1 ml of PBS (1–2 × 10⁷ cells/ml) (*see* **Note 26**).

2. Prepare 1 ml of 10 μM fluorescent dye (CFSE or CMTPX) solution in PBS.

3. Mix cell solution with fluorescent dye solution (1:1).

4. Incubate for 10 min at 37 °C, inverting the tube every 3 min (*see* **Note 27**).

5. Add 10 ml of ice-cold 10% RPMI.

6. Centrifuge at 3000 × *g* for 3 min at 4 °C and discard supernatant.

7. Wash cells as in **steps 5** and **6**.

8. Count cells.

9. Resuspend in 300 μl of 2% RPMI.

3.2.5 Adoptive Transfer of T Cells Via Tail Vein

1. Heat the recipient mice with a heating lamp for 5 min (*see* **Note 28**).

2. Fix the mice using a mouse holder.

3. Inject 300 μl of T cell suspension into the tail vein with a 30-gauge insulin syringe.

4. Proceed to the elicitation of the CHS response within 2 days.

3.2.6 Elicitation of CHS Response

1. Hold the mouse in one hand and paint 20 μl of 0.3% DNFB solution on the left ear skin (10 μl to the dorsal side and 10 μl to the ventral side) (*see* **Note 29**).

2. Air-dry the DNFB solution.

3. Set mice onto the stage and commence imaging (*see* Subheading 3.1) (Fig. 4).

3.3 Visualization of Cutaneous Blood Vessels

1. Dissolve 5 mg fluorescent-labeled dextran in 300 μl sterile PBS (*see* **Note 30**).

2. Slowly inject the dextran solution via the tail vein (*see* **Note 31**) (Fig. 5).

4 Notes

1. The skin immune response may be influenced by the hair cycle. For example, the CHS response is suppressed in the anagen (hair-growth) phase. To avoid this, the sensitization of CHS

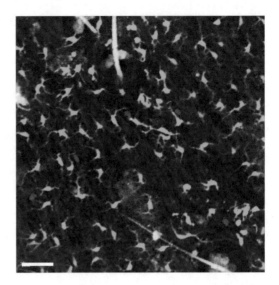

Fig. 4 Sample image. Skin-infiltrating T cells (red) interact with Langerhans cells (green). Scale bar = 50 μm

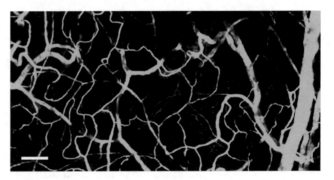

Fig. 5 Sample image. Images were acquired 10 min after 150-kDa FITC-conjugated dextran injection. Scale bar = 100 μm

should be completed within the first telogen (resting) phase (6–8 weeks after birth).

2. The skin immune response may vary among mouse strains. For example, the CHS response is stronger in BALB/c mice than C57BL/6 mice.

3. Melanin granules scatter the laser and produce strong autofluorescence. In addition, they may cause heat damage to the tissues. Therefore, albino mice are better suited for skin imaging.

4. An inverted microscope is better suited for observation of the skin than an upright microscope because of the ease of fixing the ear.

5. Hair removal cream for humans is suitable.

Table 2
Standard hapten application for the CHS response

	Sensitization			Elicitation		
	Concentration (%)	Solvent	Dose (µl)	Concentration (%)	Solvent	Dose (µl)
DNFB	0.5	Acetone:Olive oil (4:1)	25	0.3	Acetone:Olive oil (4:1)	20
TNCB	7.0	Acetone:Olive oil (4:1)	100	1.0	Acetone:Olive oil (9:1)	20
Oxazolone	3.0	100% EtOH	150	1.0	100% EtOH	20
FITC	0.5	Acetone:Dibutyl phthalate (1:1)	400	0.5	Acetone:Dibutyl phthalate (1:1)	20

DNFB 2,4-dinitrofluorobenzene, *TNCB* 2,4,6-trinitrochlorobenzene, *FITC* fluorescein isothiocyanate

6. The anesthesia is maintained for 1–1.5 h with intraperitoneal administration of pentobarbital sodium. Anesthetic gases such as isoflurane are suitable for longer anesthesia.

7. A variety of haptens are used for the induction of the CHS response. The standard hapten application chart is shown in Table 2.

8. A CD4⁺ T cell isolation kit, CD8⁺ T cell isolation kit, and CD90.2 microbeads are also available.

9. The body temperature of the mouse will drop, particularly after the anesthesia. Keep the mouse on a heating pad and warm it sufficiently. Body temperature significantly affects mouse survival and cell dynamics.

10. Ensure that the hair removal cream does not stay on the ear for more than 5 min. The cream is stimulative and may modify skin inflammation.

11. Handle the ear gently to prevent injuries arising from friction.

12. Avoid the formation of bubbles when immersion oil is placed between the objective lens and the cover glass.

13. Do not apply strong pressure to the ear as it may disturb blood and lymph circulation, which are important for intravital imaging studies.

14. The flow rate of isoflurane must be increased depending on the body weight of the mouse. Mice under good anesthesia will have a quite rapid breathing speed (not deep).

15. We observed that labeled effector T cells started to appear in the dermis within 6 h post-elicitation and formed clusters with EYFP⁺ dermal dendritic cells. The clusters became larger and

more evident after 24 h [6]. For long-time imaging (5 h~), inject PBS (~500 μl) subcutaneously to avoid dehydration.

16. Immune responses, including the CHS response, may be suppressed in stressed mice. Mice should be accustomed to their housing before sensitization.

17. The specific gravity of DNFB is 1.482 g/cm³. To prepare 6 ml of 0.5% DNFB solution, mix 20 μl of DNFB with 4.8 ml acetone and 1.2 ml olive oil.

18. Care should be taken not to damage the skin during shaving.

19. Paint DNFB solution on the center of the abdomen in a coin-sized area (Fig. 2).

20. We generally use five sensitized mice for transferring the sensitized T cells into one recipient mouse.

21. The number of DNFB-sensitized T cells in the draining lymph nodes reaches a peak at 5 or 6 days post-sensitization.

22. The draining lymph nodes of the abdominal skin are the axillary and inguinal lymph nodes. If mice are sensitized on the ear skin or the back skin, collect the auricular or brachial lymph nodes, respectively.

23. Approximately 10^8 cells can be harvested from the draining lymph nodes of five sensitized mice.

24. Separate T cells manually with MACS columns or automatically with an autoMACS pro separator.

25. Approximately $1.0–2.0 \times 10^7$ T cells are harvested from the draining lymph nodes of five sensitized mice. Note that not all T cells are DNFB-specific T cells. If necessary, keep a 50 μl aliquot for flow cytometry to ensure the purity of T cells.

26. Cells should be labeled in medium without FCS. FCS significantly interferes with the linkage of fluorescent dye to the cells.

27. Cover the heater or tube with aluminum foil to protect against light. Do not exceed 10 min since the fluorescent dye solution is cell toxic.

28. Use Langerin-eGFP mice if the interaction between T cells and epidermal Langerhans cells is the target of observation.

29. To prepare 5 ml of 0.3% DNFB solution, mix 10 μl of DNFB with 4 ml acetone and 1 ml olive oil.

30. The retention time of dextran in the blood depends on the size of dextran. In the inflammatory state, dextran immediately leaks to the extravascular space regardless of its size.

31. Blood vessels will be visualized immediately after dextran injection.

Acknowledgement

This work was supported by Grants-in-Aid for Scientific Research from the Ministry of Education, Culture, Sports, Science and Technology of Japan.

References

1. Denk W, Strickler JH, Webb WW (1990) Two-photon laser scanning fluorescence microscopy. Science 248(4951):73–76

2. Kabashima K, Egawa G (2014) Intravital multi-photon imaging of cutaneous immune responses. J Invest Dermatol 134(11):2680–2684

3. Kaplan DH, Igyártó BZ, Gaspari AA (2012) Early immune events in the induction of allergic contact dermatitis. Nat Rev Immunol 12(2):114–124

4. Honda T, Egawa G, Grabbe S, Kabashima K (2013) Update of immune events in the murine contact hypersensitivity model: toward the understanding of allergic contact dermatitis. J Invest Dermatol 133(2):303–315

5. Cahalan MD, Parker I, Wei SH, Miller MJ (2002) Two-photon tissue imaging: seeing the immune system in a fresh light. Nat Rev Immunol 2(11):872–880

6. Natsuaki Y, Egawa G, Nakamizo S, Ono S, Hanakawa S, Okada T, Kusuba N, Otsuka A, Kitoh A, Honda T (2014) Perivascular leuko-cyte clusters are essential for efficient activation of effector T cells in the skin. Nat Immunol 15(11):1064–1069

7. Okabe M, Ikawa M, Kominami K, Nakanishi T, Nishimune Y (1997) Green mice' as a source of ubiquitous green cells. FEBS Lett 407(3): 313–319

8. Tomura M, Yoshida N, Tanaka J, Karasawa S, Miwa Y, Miyawaki A, Kanagawa O (2008) Monitoring cellular movement in vivo with photoconvertible fluorescence protein "Kaede" transgenic mice. Proc Natl Acad Sci U S A 105(31):10871–10876. https://doi.org/10.1073/pnas.0802278105

9. Nowotschin S, Hadjantonakis AK (2009) Use of KikGR a photoconvertible green-to-red flu-orescent protein for cell labeling and lineage analysis in ES cells and mouse embryos. BMC Dev Biol 9:49. https://doi.org/10.1186/1471-213X-9-49

10. Celli S, Albert ML, Bousso P (2011) Visualizing the innate and adaptive immune responses underlying allograft rejection by two-photon microscopy. Nat Med 17(6):744–749

11. Kissenpfennig A, Henri S, Dubois B, Laplace-Builhé C, Perrin P, Romani N, Tripp CH, Douillard P, Leserman L, Kaiserlian D (2005) Dynamics and function of Langerhans cells in vivo: dermal dendritic cells colonize lymph node are as distinct from slower migrating Langerhans cells. Immunity 22(5):643–654

12. Abtin A, Jain R, Mitchell AJ, Roediger B, Brzoska AJ, Tikoo S, Cheng Q, Ng LG, Cavanagh LL, von Andrian UH (2014) Perivascular macrophages mediate neutrophil recruitment during bacterial skin infection. Nat Immunol 15(1):45–53

13. Matsushima H, Ogawa Y, Miyazaki T, Tanaka H, Nishibu A, Takashima A (2010) Intravital imaging of IL-1β production in skin. J Invest Dermatol 130(6):1571–1580

14. Dudeck A, Dudeck J, Scholten J, Petzold A, Surianarayanan S, Köhler A, Peschke K, Vöhringer D, Waskow C, Krieg T (2011) Mast cells are key promoters of contact allergy that mediate the adjuvant effects of haptens. Immunity 34(6):973–984

15. Gray EE, Suzuki K, Cyster JG (2011) Cutting edge: identification of a motile IL-17–produc-ing γδ T cell population in the dermis. J Immunol 186(11):6091–6095

16. Prinz I, Sansoni A, Kissenpfennig A, Ardouin L, Malissen M, Malissen B (2006) Visualization of the earliest steps of γδ T cell development in the adult thymus. Nat Immunol 7(9):995–1003

17. Hillen F, Kaijzel EL, Castermans K, oude Egbrink MG, Lowik CW, Griffioen AW (2008) A transgenic Tie2-GFP athymic mouse model; a tool for vascular biology in xenograft tumors. Biochem Biophys Res Commun 368(2):364–367. https://doi.org/10.1016/j.bbrc.2008.01.080

18. Choi I, Chung HK, Ramu S, Lee HN, Kim KE, Lee S, Yoo J, Choi D, Lee YS, Aguilar B (2011) Visualization of lymphatic vessels by Prox1-promoter directed GFP reporter in a bacterial artificial chromosome-based transgenic mouse. Blood 117(1):362–365

19. Feng G, Mellor RH, Bernstein M, Keller-Peck C, Nguyen QT, Wallace M, Nerbonne JM, Lichtman JW, Sanes JR (2000) Imaging neuro-nal subsets in transgenic mice expressing multiple spectral variants of GFP. Neuron 28(1):41–51

Chapter 9

Imaging of Inflammatory Responses in the Mouse Ear Skin

Jackson LiangYao Li, Chi Ching Goh, and Lai Guan Ng

Abstract

The skin is one of the most physiologically important organs where the organism comes into contact with the external environment and is often a site where pathogen entry first occurs. Thus, a better understanding of the specialized cellular behavior of the immune system in the skin may be important for the improved treatment of diseases. Here, we describe in detail a procedure to image the dorsal mouse ear skin, using a customized ear stage and its associated coverslip holder, with an upright multiphoton microscope. As a demonstrative example, we describe the specific protocol for visualizing robust neutrophil trafficking in albino lysozyme-EGFP mice in response to zymosan particles. Instructive sections are provided for the mouse ear preparation, intradermal delivery of zymosan, design and use of the custom ear stage, as well as a solution for the uninterrupted live imaging of mice during prolonged sessions within a dark box. The mouse ear is easily accessible for imaging, and unlike most other organs, does not require any invasive surgery to be performed.

Key words In vivo imaging, Mouse, Ear, Skin, Inflammation, Immune system

1 Introduction

In vertebrates, the skin acts as one of the first barriers between the organism and its external environment, providing primarily protection of the organism's internal organs from physical and chemical attack, as well as preventing excessive water loss [1]. Concomitant with its physical protective roles, the skin acts as the first line of immunological defense against pathogens [2], containing a wide variety of cell types that can act as immune sentinels to rapidly detect and trigger the appropriate immune responses to the specific pathogens [3]. In addition, the skin immune system also reacts to non-microbial danger signals (e.g., in the context of sterile injuries and autoimmune diseases) [4], as well as plays an important role in the prevention of skin cancers [5]. Thus, the immune system in the skin is relevant in many contexts of disease and is an attractive target for research.

Masaru Ishii (ed.), *Intravital Imaging of Dynamic Bone and Immune Systems: Methods and Protocols*, Methods in Molecular Biology, vol. 1763, https://doi.org/10.1007/978-1-4939-7762-8_9, © Springer Science+Business Media, LLC 2018

The skin has several unique characteristics that make it advantageous for intravital imaging [6]. This is especially true for the mouse ear skin. For example, the skin in the mouse ear is generally thinner than at other sites [7], allowing for the full depth of dermis to be imaged within the technical and practical limits of multiphoton microscopy. The cartilage in the mouse pinna is flexible and elastic, which allows the ear to be easily manipulated and laid flat on the stage. The distal nature of the mouse ear also means that it is easier to isolate and stabilize, avoiding the undesired vibrations arising from the mouse breathing motions and heartbeat. Because the skin is already exposed to the external environment, there is no need to perform any invasive surgical procedures, which may otherwise disrupt the normal physiology of the mouse and lead to potentially misleading interpretations of the experiments. Hence, the mouse ear skin model is uniquely suited for intravital imaging and will likely continue to be an important tool for the researcher.

Here, we provide a multiphoton microscopy imaging procedure for the dorsal mouse ear skin using a customized ear stage setup. As a robust demonstrative starting example for beginners, we describe the specific protocol for visualizing neutrophil trafficking in fluorescent reporter mice in response to relatively low-cost and commercially available preparations of yeast-derived zymosan particles. Various aspects of the imaging procedure, unique to the mouse ear imaging procedure, are detailed as a useful reference for the user. These include the mouse ear preparation, intradermal delivery of zymosan, design and use of the custom ear stage, as well as a solution for an uninterrupted imaging session that is also compatible with the use of a dark box. We anticipate that once users have mastered these basic techniques, they will be able to easily modify the procedure for answering other specific questions of interest in skin biology.

2 Materials

2.1 Mouse

1. 6–15 weeks old male or female Lysozyme-GFP albino mice. Mice are obtained by crossing lysozyme-EGFP C57BL/6 (Lyz2[tm1.1Graf], Thomas Graf, Center for Genomic Regulation, Spain) [8] onto albino C57BL/6 background (B6(Cg)-Tyr[c-2J/J], Jackson Laboratories) (see Note 1).

2.2 Anesthesia

1. Weighing balance (required calibration weight range: at least from 15 to 40 g).
2. Timer, stopwatch, or clock.
3. Integrated mouse body temperature controller, monitor, and heating pad system.
4. 30 G insulin syringe.

5. Ketamine-xylazine solution: 15 mg/mL ketamine hydrochloride, 1 mg/mL xylazine hydrochloride, in sterile water (*see* **Note 2**).

2.3 Hair Removal

1. Timer, stopwatch, or clock.

2. Integrated mouse body temperature controller, monitor, and heating pad system.

3. Medical cotton-tipped applicators.

4. Delicate task disposable wipes.

5. Depilatory cream.

6. PBS: 0.2 g/L potassium phosphate monobasic, 0.2 g/L potassium chloride, 8.0 g/L sodium chloride, 1.15 g/L sodium phosphate dibasic (anhydrous) in sterile water.

2.4 Intradermal and Intravenous Injection

1. Laboratory vacuum pump.

2. Hamilton syringe 62RN, with Hamilton needle, 33 G, length: 0.5 in., point style: 4, hub: small RN. Attach a clean Hamilton needle to a clean Hamilton syringe. Remove the plunger from the Hamilton syringe. Use a laboratory vacuum pump to extract a small amount of sterile water into the bore of the Hamilton syringe. Replace the plunger, which should now be air-tight (*see* **Note 3**).

3. Surgical stereoscopic dissecting microscope.

4. Scissors.

5. Curved forceps.

6. Medical cotton-tipped applicators.

7. 25 mL serological pipette.

8. Masking tape (approximately 2 cm wide).

9. 30 G insulin syringe.

10. Laboratory vortex mixer.

11. Cell strainer (40 μm pore size).

12. Zymosan suspension: 1 mg/mL Zymosan A from *Saccharomyces cerevisiae* in PBS. Vortex for at least 2 min at maximum speed after reconstitution in PBS, then immediately filter the suspension through a cell strainer.

13. Evans blue: 10 mg/mL in PBS.

2.5 Ear Stage Placement

1. Integrated mouse body temperature controller, monitor, and heating pad system.

2. Custom ear stage, with metal spacer clip of approximately 0.5–0.8 mm thickness (Fig. 1).

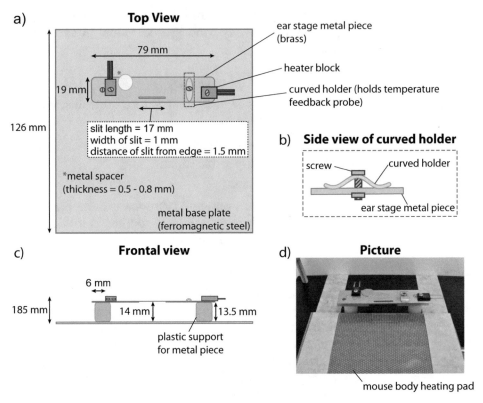

Fig. 1 Design of mouse ear stage. (**a**) Top view of stage. (**b**) Side view of the curved holder, which is used for holding the temperature feedback probe of the mouse ear stage heating system. (**c**) Frontal view of stage, showing the dimensions of the plastic supports that insulate the metal piece from the base plate. Note also the thinned portion of the metal piece at the slit region. (**d**) Photograph of the elevated ear stage portion, with the mouse body heating pad also shown

3. Integrated ear stage temperature controller, monitor, and heater blocks system (e.g., from Warner Instruments (Harvard Apparatus)).

4. High vacuum grease.

5. Cover glass (22 mm × 32 mm).

6. Custom coverslip holder and stand (Fig. 2). Attach the cover glass to coverslip holder using some high vacuum grease.

7. Scissors.

8. Curved forceps.

9. Masking tape (approximately 2 cm wide).

10. Small spring-loaded clips ×2.

11. Fine-tipped paintbrush.

12. Medical cotton-tipped applicators.

13. PBS.

Side view   **Top view**

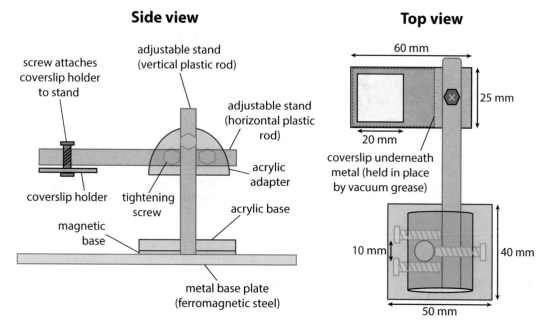

Fig. 2 Design of the coverslip holder. The coverslip holder has a magnetic base to provide firm support when placed on the metal base plate. The coverslip (22 mm × 32 mm) is held to the underside of the coverslip holder by vacuum grease and directly rests on the mouse ear during imaging. The use of a coverslip holder greatly keeps the mouse ear flat during imaging and greatly stabilizes the physical setup

2.6 In Vivo
Multiphoton Imaging

1. Sterile water.

2. PBS.

3. 2× diluted ketamine-xylazine solution: Add an equal volume of ketamine-xylazine solution to PBS (*see* **Note 4**).

4. Syringes with attached polypropylene tubing ×3. To prepare the syringes, attach 1 mL Luer disposable syringes to Luer-compatible adapters and polypropylene tubing (diameter of 1/16″ or smaller) of the appropriate length. Choose a length of tubing such that the tubing can comfortably reach its intended location from outside the dark box, but keep in mind that the longer the tubing, the larger the volume of dead space introduced, which will result in larger required volumes of prepared solutions. An optional Luer-compatible four-way stopcock placed between the syringe and polypropylene tubing will make it easy to remove air from the syringe during preparation. Fill the syringes with water, PBS or 2× diluted ketamine-xylazine solution as appropriate. Remove any air bubbles from the syringes, tubing, and needles.

5. Luer-compatible hypodermic 30 G needle. Attach this needle to the syringe with attached polypropylene tubing containing 2× diluted ketamine-xylazine solution.

6. Bench pipette (200 μL) and compatible tips.

7. Upright multiphoton microscope (capable of emitting laser pulses at 950 nm), with the following optical filter sets: 495 long-pass (LP), 560 LP, 475/42 band-pass (BP) (Second harmonic generation channel), 525/50 BP (EGFP channel), and 665/40 BP (Evans blue channel).

8. Masking tape.

9. Strings or elastic bands.

10. Fine strips of masking tape. Cut several small slices of masking tape approximately 5 mm in width and 2 cm in length. You can do this easily by cutting perpendicularly along the length of a reel of masking tape approximately 2 cm wide.

3   Methods

3.1   Mouse Anesthesia

1. Weigh and anesthetize the mouse by intraperitoneal injection of ketamine-xylazine solution (8 μL/g body weight) (*see* **Note 5**). Set a timer to keep track of the timings for anesthesia (*see* **Note 6**). Place the mouse on a heating pad to maintain its body temperature at 37 °C throughout the imaging procedure. Position the mouse such that the belly of the mouse is touching the heating pad, its head is upright (resting on its chin) and its ears are not being folded or touching the heating pad (*see* **Note 7**).

3.2   Mouse Ear Hair Removal

1. Using cotton tip applicators, apply a moderate amount (*see* **Note 8**) of depilatory cream to the mouse ear to be imaged, ensuring that at least two thirds of the mouse ear (from the edges) are fully covered (*see* **Note 9**). Take no more than 30 s to finish performing this action.

2. Wait for three more minutes, paying particular attention to the timing (*see* **Note 10**).

3. Dip several (about 6–10) cotton tip applicators into PBS, and use these wet cotton tip applicators to remove the depilatory cream from the mouse ear (*see* **Note 11**). Be gentle, but thorough, paying particular attention to the edge of the ear. Do not contaminate the PBS, e.g., by reusing the cotton tip applicators, especially if they have touched the depilatory cream.

4. Use a piece of delicate disposable wipes to very gently dry the ears by blotting. Both sides of the ears need to be dry, not just the dorsal side (*see* **Note 12**). Allow the ears to air dry for at least another 20 s thereafter.

3.3   Injection of Zymosan and Evans Blue Dye

1. Prepare a 25 mL serological pipette as the base for intradermal injection. Cut a 12–15 cm piece of masking tape. By holding one end of the tape, paste the masking tape on to the center of the serological pipette, such that the tape is exactly 90° to the

length of the serological pipette, using the markings on the serological pipette as a guide. Then, wrap the masking tape approximately one time around the serological pipette. Next, by reversing the direction of rotation, wrap the rest of the masking tape tightly around itself (*see* **Note 13**), such that the sticky side now faces outwards (Fig. 3).

2. Position the serological pipette with the ring of masking tape under a dissecting microscope, and adjust the magnification (use a 40× objective if possible) and focus as necessary.

3. Position the mouse such that the ventral part of its ear lies very close to the ring of masking tape. Then, using two cotton tip applicators, gently press down on the mouse ear such that it sticks to the masking tape. Do not allow the mouse ear to become folded, and avoid letting the hair from the mouse head from touching the masking tape. Adjust the mouse ear and serological pipette as necessary such that the targeted injection site is comfortably centered in the field of view under the dissecting microscope and is in focus. The injection site should ideally be approximately 1.5 mm away from the furthermost edge of the ear, avoiding the major visible vessels. Lock down the position by firmly taping down both ends of the serological pipette to the table (*see* **Note 14**) (Fig. 4).

4. Vortex the zymosan suspension thoroughly at maximum speed for at least 20 s. Load the Hamilton syringe with 1.0 µL of zymosan suspension (*see* **Note 15**). Bend the needle of the Hamilton syringe slightly (in the direction of the bevel).

5. Rest the needle of the Hamilton syringe on the dorsal mouse ear skin at the targeted site of injection, with the bevel facing upwards (*see* **Note 16**). While looking through the dissecting microscope, raise the barrel of the Hamilton syringe such that the bevel is approximately 45° from the ear surface, and gently pierce the mouse skin surface with the needle. The needle should only penetrate approximately one-quarter the length of the bevel. Then, carefully lower the barrel of the syringe such that the bevel is now approximately 25° to the skin surface. Now, further penetrate the needle into the skin such that the bevel is just fully covered (*see* **Note 17**). Holding the needle steady, slowly inject the contents of the syringe into the skin by pushing the plunger (*see* **Note 18**). The ear tissue should swell at the injection site as the contents are delivered, indicating a successful injection. If the skin does not swell, the needle has most likely penetrated too far past both the cartilage and the ventral skin (*see* **Note 19**) (Fig. 5).

6. Scruff the mouse by the base of its neck, and gently remove the mouse ear from the masking tape by lifting the head of the mouse away from the masking tape, taking care not to injure the mouse ear (*see* **Note 20**).

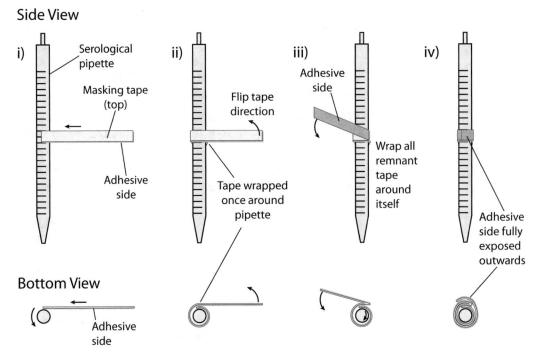

Fig. 3 Preparation of the serological pipette and masking tape for stable intradermal injections. The steps for applying the masking tape to the 25 mL serological pipette are shown. The end result is a ring of masking tape pasted to the serological pipette with its adhesive side exposed outwards in all directions

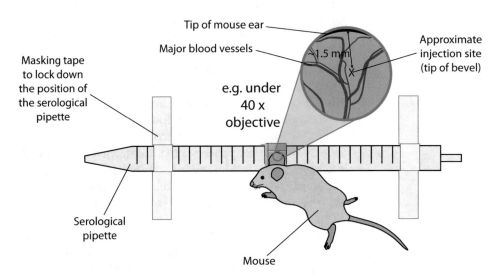

Fig. 4 Placement of the mouse ear, masking tapes, and serological pipette for intradermal injections. The position of the serological pipette and mouse ear has to be locked down by a masking tape on each end of the pipette once the desired injection spot is identified under the dissecting microscope. The approximate ideal injection spot is also demonstrated in the figure

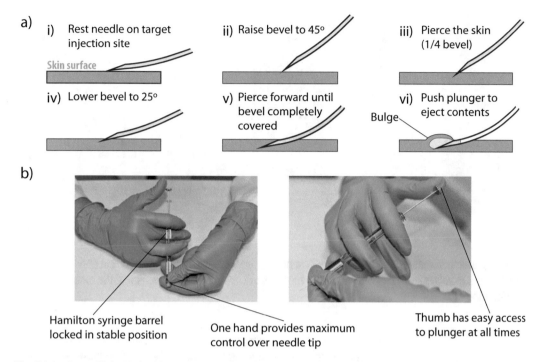

Fig. 5 Intradermal injection with 2.5 μL Hamilton syringe. (**a**) Sequential steps showing the intradermal injection are shown. A successful injection will result in a bulge containing the delivered liquid contents. (**b**) Suggested method of holding Hamilton syringe while performing intradermal injection

7. Inject Evans blue dye intravenously into the mouse (2 μL/g body weight) (*see* **Note 21**).

3.4 Ear Placement on Ear Stage

1. Cut a piece of masking tape approximately 5 cm in length. Using forceps to manipulate the masking tape, fold the masking tape on itself such that approximately 2 cm of the adhesive side of the masking tape adheres to another 2 cm of the adhesive side, leaving behind only approximately 1 cm of the adhesive portion exposed. Trim the masking tape to size (about 0.8 cm width × 1.5 cm length) such that only about 1 mm of the adhesive portion of the masking tape is exposed (*see* **Note 22**). Insert this masking tape about halfway through the slit of the mouse ear stage, with the exposed adhesive side facing the heating pad, and positioned below the metal piece of the mouse ear stage (Fig. 6).

2. Position the mouse ear close to the masking tape strip. Using one hand, place a cotton tip applicator behind the exposed adhesive area of the masking tape strip to act as a bracing support. Then, using another cotton tip applicator with the other hand, gently press the mouse ear against the exposed adhesive area so that the ventral mouse ear sticks to the masking tape strip. There should be an approximately 4 mm distance between the tip of the mouse ear and the region of adhesion (*see* **Note 23**).

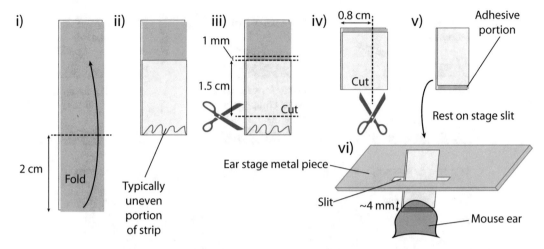

Fig. 6 Preparation of masking tape strip for pulling mouse ear through ear stage slit. The sequence of steps for preparing the masking tape strip is shown. Also shown is the approximate positioning of the mouse ear on the masking tape strip

3. Using a pair of forceps to hold on to the masking tape, carefully guide the mouse ear through the slit (*see* **Note 24**) while simultaneously moving the mouse body, such that the mouse ear does not experience excessive tension from being pulled through the slit. After the ear has been pulled through, allow the masking tape to rest on the metal piece by its weight. Do not allow the mouse ear to fold upon itself (*see* **Note 25**) (Fig. 7).

4. Clamp the masking tape strip on to the metal piece of the mouse ear stage, using two spring-loaded clips (*see* **Note 26**). Wet a fine-tipped paintbrush with PBS, and gently but forcefully insert the bristles between the ventral mouse ear and masking tape strip, making sure to fully wet the adhesive portion of the masking tape strip (*see* **Note 27**). At this point, the masking tape strip should have lost its adhesiveness completely. Remove the spring-loaded clips, and using a pair of forceps, pull out the masking tape strip from under the mouse ear in the direction away from the mouse head (Fig. 8).

5. Using cotton tip applicators, gently flatten the mouse ear over the ear stage metal piece. The ear should be able to be stably held to the ear stage metal piece by water tension from the PBS earlier deposited by the paintbrush. However, if the area under the mouse ear is too dry, the ear may not stay in place. In this case, lift up the mouse ear using the cotton tip applicators and place a small drop of PBS under the mouse ear before flattening the mouse ear again (*see* **Note 28**).

6. Using a pipette, place a small drop of PBS (approximately 30 μL) on the dorsal mouse ear over the intended imaging

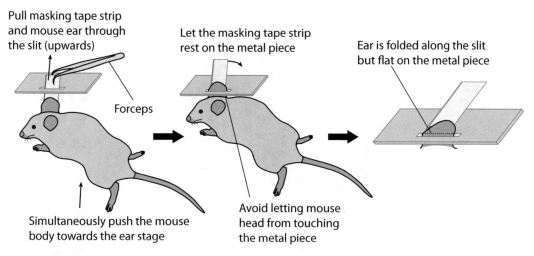

Fig. 7 Getting the mouse ear through the ear stage slit. The sequence of steps for pulling the mouse ear through the slit using the masking tape strip is shown

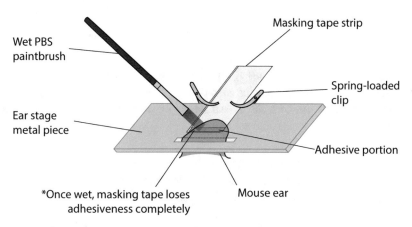

Fig. 8 Removal of mouse ear from masking tape strip. The figure shows the location of the spring-loaded clips relative to the masking tape strip. Once the masking tape strip is firmly secured, using a wet paintbrush to remove the adhesiveness of the masking tape strip becomes very easy, and allows for the gentle release of the mouse ear with minimal injury

spot (where the zymosan suspension was injected). Surface tension should hold the droplet in place, but if the dorsal ear was previously wet, or if too much PBS was placed, the PBS droplet may break and get drawn under the mouse ear. In this case, dry the dorsal ears carefully with delicate disposable wipes, and repeat the placement of the PBS droplet on the dorsal mouse ear. Place a second droplet of PBS under the coverslip attached to the coverslip holder.

7. Lower the coverslip over the mouse ear and allow the two PBS droplets to merge (*see* **Note 29**). Lower the coverslip holder

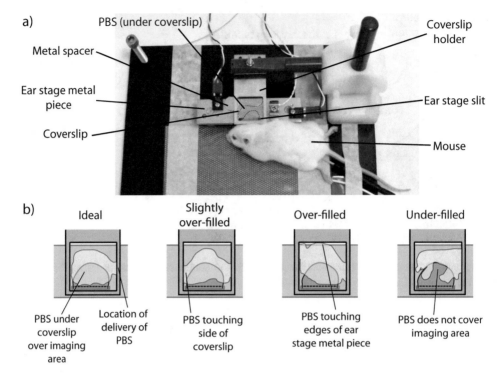

Fig. 9 Setup of mouse ear stage before imaging. (**a**) The photograph demonstrates how the mouse ear stage is to be finally set up, just before connecting the optional syringes and tubing. (**b**) Schematic diagram demonstrates where the PBS under the coverslip should ideally be located for a successfully stable imaging session

to its minimum height such that the coverslip rests on the metal spacer, and the mouse ear is just under very slight pressure from the coverslip (*see* **Note 30**) (Fig. 9).

3.5 Imaging

1. Place the mouse ear stage on to the microscope stage such that the coverslip is directly under the microscope objective. Move the mouse and ear stage such that they are as close to the final imaging position as possible (*see* **Note 31**).

2. Following manufacturer instructions, connect up all the wires as necessary for maintaining the ear stage at 35 °C (*see* **Note 32**). This typically includes connecting up the electrical wires to the heater blocks of the mouse ear stage, as well as the feedback temperature probe for the mouse ear stage.

3. Following manufacturer instructions, connect up all the wires as necessary for maintaining the body temperature of the mouse at 37 °C. This typically includes connecting up the electrical wires of the mouse heating pad to the power box, as well as inserting the rectal temperature probe into the mouse.

4. Secure all loose wires with masking tape, ensuring that none of the wires are under any significant tension (*see* **Note 33**).

5. Using a few pieces of strings/elastic bands and masking tape, secure the flexible tubing of the syringe containing water to the microscope objective, such that water will flow directly from the mouth of the tubing to under the microscope objective when ejected from the syringe (*see* **Note 34**).

6. Similarly, using fine strips of masking tape, secure the flexible tubing of the syringe containing PBS to the mouse ear stage such that PBS will be able to flow from the mouth of the tubing to directly under the coverslip (*see* **Note 35**). This is achieved most easily by resting the mouth of the tubing directly flush against one edge of the coverslip holder (*see* **Note 36**).

7. Pierce the needle of the syringe containing 2× diluted ketamine-xylazine solution into the mouse back flank skin in a manner similar to performing a subcutaneous injection. Secure the needle to the mouse by using a fine strip of masking tape (*see* **Note 37**).

8. If necessary, carefully place the syringe barrels (water, PBS, and ketamine-xylazine solution) outside the dark box (*see* **Note 38**) and secure any loose tubing with masking tape (Fig. 10).

9. Following manufacturer instructions, set up the upright multiphoton microscope for imaging of the dorsal mouse ear skin near the region of zymosan injection. Use the Ti:Sa laser at 950 nm at an output power of approximately 30 mW for initial

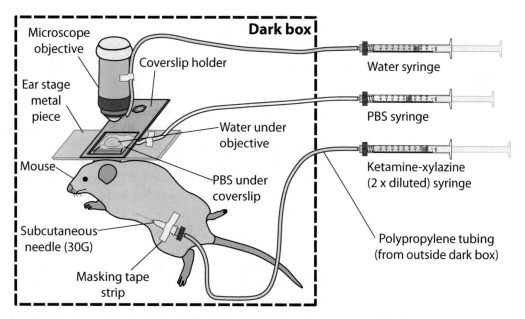

Fig. 10 Setup for continuous uninterrupted intravital imaging of mouse ear within the microscope dark box. Shown is a schematic diagram of the positioning of the syringes and tubing for the delivery of fluids necessary to ensure an uninterrupted imaging session

previewing. Slowly raise (or lower) the laser power accordingly for good image contrast, but do not raise the laser power too high as to cause heat-induced "speckling" [9] (*see* **Note 39**).

10. Locate desired imaging field of view and perform imaging of the mouse ear. Capture 450 μm × 450 μm × 60 μm ($X \times Y \times Z$) image time-lapse z-stacks, with approximately 1 min time gaps between image acquisition (*see* **Note 40**), for the desired length of time (typically 1–3 h).

11. Maintain the anesthesia on the mouse by injecting the ketamine-xylazine solution using the syringe from outside the dark box (after the initial hour, 4 μL/g body weight, once every half hour thereafter) (*see* **Note 41**). Top up the PBS under the coverslip (lost to evaporation) by injecting approximately 20 μL every 20 min (*see* **Note 42**). Similarly, top up the water under the objective by injecting approximately 30 μL every hour. If done correctly, there should not be any need to interrupt the imaging, with the exception of z-drifts due to the ear swelling from the inflammation (*see* **Note 43**). Evans blue dye contrast may be degraded rapidly over time due to vascular leakage.

12. At the end of the imaging session, dismantle all the wires and tubes as appropriate. Remove the mouse from the ear stage and sacrifice the mouse according to institutional guidelines.

13. Visualize and analyze the imaging results as appropriate using the relevant software (e.g., ImageJ). GFP-positive neutrophils should be observed actively swarming into the interstitium of the mouse ear from the medium-sized venules (*see* **Note 44**).

4 Notes

1. In these mice, cells of the monomyelocytic lineage express EGFP, and include neutrophils (very high EGFP expression levels), monocytes, and macrophages (low EGFP expression levels) [10]. It is highly recommended that mice are converted to an albino background because this greatly reduces the likelihood of heat injury resulting from the "speckling" phenomenon [9].

2. Drugs will gradually lose efficacy over time. It is recommended to always prepare the drugs fresh since the loss of drug efficacy may result in a loss of temporal control over the dosing anesthesia by the user. Do not use drugs which have been prepared more than a week ago.

3. Also ensure that the needle and syringe have been properly tightened such that it is air-tight. You can test this by sucking up water through the assembled syringe and needle (without

the plunger). Place the needle such that only its bevel is submerged under water. While sucking water up from the other end, there should be no bubbles appearing in the bore of the syringe. This is potentially critical since the syringe calibration would become inaccurate, and the volumes of zymosan injected would become inconsistent between experiments.

4. Diluting the ketamine-xylazine solution with PBS reduces wastage of the drugs arising from the dead space of the syringe. It also helps to hydrate the mouse during the imaging session.

5. Correct dosing of the anesthesia is critical in any imaging experiment, as mistakes almost always lead to premature termination of the experiment, e.g., insufficient anesthesia may lead to the mouse waking up and pulling their ears out of the ear stage, whereas excessive anesthesia may lead to premature mouse death. Since drug effectiveness may vary according to location, manufacturer, and mice strains, some familiarization and optimization with the dosages may be necessary. For example, as a gauge, our mice almost always fall into deep anesthesia within 4 min if left undisturbed immediately after injection.

6. In our experience, researchers often forget to reset the timers after injecting the first follow-up dose, thereby leading to loss of control over the subsequent anesthesia. Hence, it is recommended to record down either the actual exact (clock) timings of injection or to use a count-up timer (i.e., without alarm).

7. Do not injure the mouse ears prematurely. This warning is applicable throughout the whole procedure, e.g., during scruffing or intravenous injections whereby the researcher may tend to inadvertently contort the mouse ears in order to get a firmer grip, etc.

8. By "moderate" amount, we mean that the depilatory cream should be fully covering the mouse hairs, but the mouse hairs beneath the cream should still be vaguely visible (i.e., layer of depilatory cream should be sufficiently thin as to be translucent, not opaque white). In our experience, although we are unsure of the cause, excessive cream application actually seems to *reduce* its effectiveness, possibly due to the need for optimal pH adjustment by air.

9. Although only a very small part of the ear will likely be imaged, it is still necessary to remove the rest of the hair, since mouse hair is naturally waterproof, and may cause problems later with the PBS retention under the coverslip.

10. Do not allow the depilatory cream to stay on the skin for too long, as it can cause skin inflammation and irritation if it penetrates deep into the dermis.

11. Use cotton tip applicators which are as wet as possible (i.e., dripping wet). This ensures that any remnant acids or alkalis

(from the depilatory cream) are fully neutralized. The copious amount of PBS also makes it much easier to remove the fallen hairs, reducing the likelihood that unwanted stray hairs become trapped under the coverslip, and impede the microscope laser.

12. Any moisture on the mouse ventral skin will reduce the adhesiveness of the masking tape in the next steps.

13. If the tape is not wrapped around itself tightly enough, the adhesive surface will end up being highly uneven, which may make the subsequent intradermal injection much more difficult.

14. Stabilizing the serological pipette is a very important step critical to the success of the intradermal injection. A countering force is necessary for the needle to successfully pierce through the skin when the needle force is applied. For convenience, the two masking tapes used to lock down the position can be substituted by two heavy pieces of metal weights (e.g., 0.5 kg) that can press down on the serological pipette. Friction pads on the weights also may be necessary to prevent the serological pipette from rolling. Alternatively, getting help from a colleague to hold down the serological pipette from the sides during the intradermal injection is also a possible solution.

15. Ensure that the zymosan suspension is as homogeneous as possible since large clumps of zymosan may cause the high gauge needle to become occluded.

16. Using two hands to hold the syringe, and resting the elbows on the table, or against the edge of the table will likely prevent the hands from shaking, and thus aid the stabilization of the needle during the injection.

17. The bevel needs to be fully covered by the skin in order to deposit its contents when the barrel plunger is pushed. If incomplete, the fluid will simply flow out from the region of least resistance (i.e., the air) and onto the skin surface. On the other hand, do not push the needle bevel too far in, as the physical injury due to the needle may become too large. There is also a high risk of the bevel penetrating to the other side of the ear.

18. The needle bevel needs to be held steady during this step. Otherwise, there is a risk of enlarging the injury site more than necessary. Attempt to hold the needle in a way such that the thumb always has ready access to the plunger (Fig. 5b).

19. If this happens, you may want to repeat the procedure on another mouse. However, if you wish to continue with imaging the same mouse, choose another spot relatively far away from the initial injury to attempt the intradermal injection again. This is because if the cavities created by the two needle injections happen to merge, the fluid will flow out from the exit created by the first injection.

20. Resist the temptation to use cotton tip applicators to remove the mouse ear away from the masking tape. Doing so almost always results in damage to the mouse ear, especially at its delicate edges (where imaging will be carried out). Instead, pulling the whole mouse head away from the masking tape actually leads to an evenly spread pressure over the whole mouse ear, with the brunt of the forces being resisted by the thick base pinna muscles and cartilage, i.e., almost no damage to the ear.

21. Evans blue dye fluoresces only when bound to albumins present in the mouse blood plasma. The dye is very bright and easily excites over a wide range of excitation wavelengths. If necessary, you can safely increase the injection volumes by at least five times (or up to the volumes as determined by your institutional guidelines) with no apparent toxicity to the mouse (e.g., to take photographs of vascular leakage of the whole ear at the end of the experiment).

22. The reason for cutting the large masking tape strip down to size, instead of directly making the masking tape strip at its final size, is that due to the nature of the masking tape, it is difficult to exactly fold the masking tape such that the edges are exactly parallel/perpendicular. This would result in portions of the masking tape retaining their adhesive properties at unwanted locations on the sides, and these adhesive parts may cause unintended problems when attempting their removal from the ear stage later. Also, the masking tape strip would scrunch up badly at one end if it has not been perfectly folded. Simply cutting away the last parts of the masking tape strip releases the tension and results in a perfectly flat piece of masking tape strip. The thin strip of exposed adhesive (1 mm) allows the easy subsequent removal of the mouse ear from the masking tape, while still providing sufficient adhesive strength to lift the mouse ear through the mouse ear stage slit.

23. The region where the adhesive strip is applied to the mouse ear determines how easy or difficult it will be later to pull the mouse ear through the ear stage slit, as well as to remove the masking tape from the ear stage with the wet paintbrush.

24. Do not scrape the mouse ear on the edges of the ear stage slit. Ensure that the mouse ear does not touch the edges when pulling vertically through the slit. Once the mouse ear has been flattened down, do not adjust the base of the mouse ear any further, as that may cause friction at the edges.

25. If the mouse ear does become folded, try adjusting the angle that the forceps is holding the masking tape strip to release the folding. Only use forceps to unfold the mouse ear as a last resort.

26. The spring-loaded clips provide tension to counter the forces from the wet paintbrush when attempting to get the paintbrush under the mouse ear for dislodging the ear from the tape.

27. Remember that the aim here is simply to get the paintbrush under the skin (in between the skin and the masking tape) so as to wet the adhesive portion of the masking tape strip. There is no need to apply much force.

28. The droplet of PBS should stay on the metal piece with an intact surface tension. If it gets drained away to the sides, dry the metal piece, and place the water drop again. Avoid letting the droplet touch the edges of the metal piece.

29. Doing this helps to ensure that the region of interest (i.e., imaging region) is fully covered by PBS between the coverslip and mouse ear skin. Do note that occasionally, some parts of the mouse ear can trap air bubbles (as might happen if the hydrophobic depilatory cream was not fully removed, etc.), but if the region of interest is not affected, there is no need to attempt their removal.

30. The mouse ear should be under minimal pressure from the coverslip, but it should not be completely free-floating on the PBS, as drifts may occur easily later. If this is the case, the metal spacer may need to be changed to another spacer of a smaller thickness or adjusted further away from the mouse ear, depending on the rigidity of the coverslip holder.

31. By positioning the mouse as close to its final imaging position as possible, this minimizes the likelihood that some wire or tubing will later be under undue tension or be in an awkward position when the whole setup is finally moved into position.

32. The mouse ear, like other parts of its extremities, is typically a few degrees cooler than body temperature under steady state. Thus, mouse ear stage temperature is set at only 35 °C instead of at body temperature. Also, be aware that resistive heater blocks can rapidly heat the ear stage metal piece up to over 100 °C within minutes if not controlled. To prevent the mouse ear from getting burnt or injured, ensure that the feedback control thermistor has been properly secured to the ear stage before turning on the ear stage temperature controllers. Also, once the heating is turned on, ensure that the machine is correctly detecting the metal plate temperature from the feedback control thermistor (e.g., detected temperature should be slowly rising, and not stay at the room temperature for prolonged period of time if the heater blocks are working).

33. Wires under tension may cause damage to the wire itself. More importantly, it may also cause the setup to be changed when the tension is eventually slowly or suddenly released. For example, an improperly inserted rectal probe may be slowly pushing the mouse body away from the ear stage, eventually causing its mouse ear to be pulled away from the ear stage, thereby causing severe XY-drifts in the imaging area.

34. This prevents the water under the objective from drying out. However, this step is actually optional if this is not a regular problem experienced by the user.

35. This solves a problem that the user is very likely to experience, as the PBS gets evaporated from under the coverslip, especially since the metal piece is continuously being heated throughout the imaging. Note that the PBS under the coverslip should avoid being overfilled (i.e., touching the outer edges of the ear stage metal piece) (Fig. 9), e.g., which may occur if the rate of PBS top up greatly exceeds the evaporation rate. If the excess PBS drains down from the elevated ear stage, it will form a connected fluid path leading to a lower height. By water tension and gravity, this may also drain away the rest of the PBS under the coverslip, paradoxically reducing the PBS availability under the coverslip. As an alternative to using the syringe and tubing, with a pipette, the user can periodically top up the PBS under the coverslip during the gap time in between image capture (i.e., when the microscope objective is stationary). However, to prevent damage to the light-sensitive detectors and microscope, attempt this only if the imaging settings provide a sufficiently long gap time.

36. The mouth of the PBS tubing must be positioned in such a way that there is a connected fluid path for the PBS ejected from the syringe to reach the PBS in the area being imaged (by water tension). This should be tested before starting imaging by injecting a small amount of PBS and observing to see if the surface area of the PBS trapped under the coverslip increases as a result. This fluid path must not be allowed to completely dry out (e.g., which may occur if the PBS top up is too infrequent) since then further release of PBS from the syringe may not be guaranteed to reach the imaging area if the fluid path is broken.

37. This allows the mouse to be anesthetized remotely from outside the dark box without interrupting the imaging process. It also completely isolates the physical movements arising from the injection of anesthesia from reaching the mouse, thereby ensuring a stable setup. Thus, this step is highly recommended even if no dark box is used.

38. Keep careful records of the timings for each injection, as their timely delivery may be the fine line that separates a successful continuous imaging session from an irrecoverable one. These data may also greatly aid any necessary future troubleshooting with the anesthesia.

39. "Speckling" has been shown to lead to chemotactic responses by neutrophils. This may cause imaging artifacts if not carefully prevented [9].

40. The temporal resolution should be increased if the neutrophils are traveling too fast in the interstitium for cell tracking. You can either sacrifice the dwell time of the microscope laser (i.e., higher image scanning frequency), reduce the thickness of the z-stack, or reduce the spatial resolution of the images.

41. As drug efficacy may vary, there may be a need to optimize the timing of the injections. Consistency of the anesthesia can be improved by always maintaining a consistent body temperature of the mouse for every imaging session, keeping the room consistently silent (avoiding sudden loud noises which may disrupt the state of arousal of the mouse), as well as investing in remote monitoring systems of the mouse (e.g., pulse oximeter). As a general guide, the mouse should be under consistent deep anesthesia without reaching the arousal stage whereby the whiskers start to move and its breathing becomes shallow. An alternative option is to use a continuous drug delivery system, such as a syringe pump or an inhalational anesthetic system (e.g., isoflurane).

42. The rate of topping up may need to be optimized for each laboratory since the evaporation rates of water depends on several factors such as the humidity of the dark box.

43. Under severe inflammation, high levels of edema may cause the ear to swell and hence change the z-positions relative to the microscope objective. Use the autofluorescent mouse remnant hair and hair follicles as a guide to decide if the imaging needs to be interrupted and the acquisition parameters corrected. For the ease of making quick decisions during imaging, we recommend taking a snapshot or print screen image at the start of the imaging session to keep as a reference for determining the severity of the imaging drifts, if any.

44. In the mouse ear, venules and arterioles are almost always found together as a parallel or gently intertwining pair of blood vessels, radiating outwards with smaller vessels branching to the sides. The arterioles are usually easily recognized with thicker collagen, smaller diameters, and fast blood flow, whereas the venules have thinner collagen, larger diameters, and slower blood flow. Upon inflammation, neutrophils roll almost exclusively on the venules [11, 12].

Acknowledgement

This work was supported by A*STAR funding. Much of the design of the ear stage and revisions to the protocol had received contributions from multiple colleagues in Singapore Immunology Network (A*STAR), as well as various other institutes.

References

1. Wickett RR, Visscher MO (2006) Structure and function of the epidermal barrier. Am J Infect Control 34:S98–S110. https://doi.org/10.1016/j.ajic.2006.05.295

2. Nestle FO, Di Meglio P, Qin JZ, Nickoloff BJ (2009) Skin immune sentinels in health and disease. Nat Rev Immunol 9:679–691. https://doi.org/10.1038/nri2622

3. Mann ER, Smith KM, Bernardo D, Al-Hassi HO, Knight SC, Hart AL (2012) Review: skin and the immune system. J Clin Exp Dermatol Res 2:003. https://doi.org/10.4172/2155-9554.S2-003

4. Chen GY, Nunez G (2010) Sterile inflammation: sensing and reacting to damage. Nat Rev Immunol 10:826–837. https://doi.org/10.1038/nri2873

5. SH Y, Bordeaux JS, Baron ED (2014) The immune system and skin cancer. Adv Exp Med Biol 810:182–1918

6. Yew E, Rowlands C, So PT (2014) Application of multiphoton microscopy in dermatological studies: a mini-review. J Innov Opt Health Sci 7:1330010. https://doi.org/10.1142/S1793545813300103

7. Tong PL et al (2015) The skin immune atlas: three-dimensional analysis of cutaneous leukocyte subsets by multiphoton microscopy. J Invest Dermatol 135:84–93. https://doi.org/10.1038/jid.2014.289

8. Faust N, Varas F, Kelly LM, Heck S, Graf T (2000) Insertion of enhanced green fluorescent protein into the lysozyme gene creates mice with green fluorescent granulocytes and macrophages. Blood 96:719–726

9. Li JL et al (2012) Intravital multiphoton imaging of immune responses in the mouse ear skin. Nat Protoc 7:221–234. https://doi.org/10.1038/nprot.2011.438

10. von Bruhl ML et al (2012) Monocytes, neutrophils, and platelets cooperate to initiate and propagate venous thrombosis in mice in vivo. J Exp Med 209:819–835. https://doi.org/10.1084/jem.20112322

11. Goh CC et al (2015) Real-time imaging of dendritic cell responses to sterile tissue injury. J Invest Dermatol 135:1181–1184. https://doi.org/10.1038/jid.2014.506

12. Li JL et al (2016) Neutrophils self-regulate immune complex-mediated cutaneous inflammation through CXCL2. J Investig Dermatol 136:416–424. https://doi.org/10.1038/jid.2015.410

Chapter 10

In Vivo Imaging of Immune Cells in Peyer's Patches

Andrea Reboldi

Abstract

Peyer's patches (PPs) are secondary lymphoid organs that coordinate the immunoglobulin A (IgA) response against commensal and pathogenic bacteria. In contrast to the immune dynamics in peripheral lymph nodes, the dynamics of immune response in PP have not been extensively characterized in vivo by two-photon microscopy, mainly due to the PP location on the anti-mesenteric side of the small intestine and the associated peristaltic movement.

Here, we describe an approach based on a custom-made spring-loaded platform to immobilize PPs and allow for two-photon microscopy imaging in vivo. We also list different strategies based on fluorescent dyes, as well as Cre/Lox and Reporter-based system, that can be used to image specific immune cell populations in distinct areas of PPs.

Key words Peyer's patches, Spring-loaded platform, Peristaltic movement, In vivo imaging, Subepithelial dome, Follicle-associated epithelium, Interfollicular region

1 Introduction

Immune cells are constantly on the move, recirculating between blood and lymphoid organs and migrating into the tissue to assure protection and maintain homeostasis. Two-photon microscopy has been developed as a method to visualize and investigate the dynamics of the immune cells in vivo or ex vivo. Its real-time nature and its ability to visualize immune cell processes in their native anatomical location make two-photon microscopy a valuable tool to study immune dynamics that cannot be recapitulated in vitro.

Peyer's patches (PPs) are secondary lymphoid follicles distributed along the anti-mesenteric side of the small intestine: their number ranges from 100 to 200 in human and 6 to 12 in mice.

PPs are organized into three major regions: the B cell follicles, which represent 80% of PPs; the subepithelial dome (SED), which is located beneath follicle-associated epithelium (FAE); and the interfollicular region (IFR), a T cell zone adjacent to the B cell follicle.

Masaru Ishii (ed.), *Intravital Imaging of Dynamic Bone and Immune Systems: Methods and Protocols*, Methods in Molecular Biology, vol. 1763, https://doi.org/10.1007/978-1-4939-7762-8_10, © Springer Science+Business Media, LLC 2018

Each of these regions can be imaged by 2P microscopy, according to the orientation of the PP.

Among secondary lymphoid tissues, PPs are peculiar due to their continuous exposure to antigens, either food-derived or microbiome-derived [1]. For this reason, PPs are attractive lymphoid organs for imaging active immune responses without the need of immunization or pathogen infection.

PPs are home of several immune dynamics that can be investigated using 2P microscopy, including lymphocyte entry, transit, and egress [2, 3]; T cell and B cell activation [4], germinal center [5] and post-germinal center events [6], plasma cell generation [7] and antigen sampling by dendritic cells [8].

PP location represents a major challeng to imaging: the intestinal peristaltic movement can induce wide movement of the tissue, making virtually impossible to follow and quantify cell motility during time-lapse imaging. This protocol is based on the use of a custom-made spring-loaded platform to immobilize PP and control peristaltic movement that has been successfully used to image spleen [9] and small intestine [10].

2   Materials

A critical part in two-photon microscopy is the choice of the fluorophores and the microscope setting. Those are highly empirical, Note and Tables 1, 2, 3 summarize general strategies based on published data and personal experience.

Appropriate authorization for experimental surgical practice on living animals needs to be obtained from the relevant veterinary authorities of the country in which the experiment is performed. Please note that all experiments should be conducted in accordance with relevant ethics, guidelines, and regulations.

2.1 Stage   Glass coverslip (thickness: 0.15 ± 0.02 mm, dimension: 22×40 mm).

Table 1
Two-photon excitation and emission wavelengths of commonly used fluorescent proteins during two-photon microscopy

Fluorophores	Peak excitation (nm)	Emission (nm)
GFP	900–1000	510
CFP	800–900	<500
YFP	930–1000	530
dsRed/RFP	1000	580–600

Table 2
Dye-based, Cre-/Lox-based, and reporter-based strategies to visualize specific immune cells during two-photon microscopy

Cell type	Transfer	Useful dye	Useful Cre	Useful reporter
T cells	Yes	CFSE, CMTMR, CellTraceViolet	Cd4	CD2-DsRed
T reg	Yes	CFSE, CMTMR, CellTraceViolet	Foxp3	Foxp3-GFP
				Foxp3-RFP
B cell	Yes	CFSE, CMTMR, CellTraceViolet	Cd19	No
			Mb1	
Plasma cell	No	No	Prdm1	Prdm1-YFP
Dendritic cells	No	No	Itgax	Itgax-YFP
			Cx3xr1	Zbtb46-GFP
			Zbtb46	Cx3xr1-GFP
				Csfr1-GFP
				Csfr1-CFP
Macrophages	No	No	Lyz2	Lyz2-GFP
			Cx3cr1	Cx3xr1-GFP
				Csfr1-GFP
				Csfr1-CFP
Monocyte	Yes	CFSE, CMTMR, CellTraceViolet	Lyz2	Lyz2-GFP
			Cx3cr1	Cx3xr1-GFP
				Ccr2-GFP
				Ccr2-RFP
				Csfr1-GFP
				Csfr1-CFP
Neutrophils	No	No	Lyz2	Lyz2-GFP
			Cx3cr1	Cx3xr1-GFP
				Csfr1-GFP
				Csfr1-CFP
Others/all	No	No	Mx-1	Ubc-GFP
			ER	Actin-CFP
			Vav	Actin-RFP
			CMV	

Table 3
Dye-based, Cre-/Lox-based, and reporter-based strategies to visualize specific immune cells in Peyer's patches micro-anatomical niches during two-photon microscopy

Location	Transfer	Reporter/Cre
SED	No	Itgax. Cx3cr1, Csfr1
IFR	Yes	Cd2, Cd4
Follicle	Yes	Cd19, Mb1
GC	No	Aicda
Epithelium	No	Villin
M cells	No	Pgrp_S

O ring (thickness: 3 mm, diameter: 2.5 cm).

Stage (7 cm × 3.6 cm) with a central window (diameter: 2 cm) and holes (diameter: 4 mm).

Screws (2.5 cm, 3 mm thick across with a top screw).

Spring (3.5 cm).

2.2 Anesthesia

Ketamine (100 mg/ml). Ketamine is a controlled drug and all relevant local regulations should be followed.

Xylazil-20 (20 mg/ml). Xylazine is a controlled drug and all relevant local regulations should be followed.

Eye protective cream (Dexpanthenol 50 mg/g).

Optional: Fentanyl.

2.3 Surgery

Heated stage (BioTherm Micro S37, Biogenics).

0.02% chlorhexidine gluconate.

Scissors (surgical, sterile, two pairs).

Forceps (surgical, sterile).

Tissue adhesive.

2.4 Imaging

Thermoconductive putty.

Saline.

Dual temperature controller.

7MP two-photon microscope (Carl Zeiss) with a Chameleon Laser (Coherent).

2.5 Analysis

Images acquisition software (ZEN2009 Carl Zeiss).

Images analysis software (Imaris 7.4.2 × 64, Bitplane; metamorph molecular devices).

Statistical analysis software (GraphPad Prism 5.0 Sun Microsystems).

3   Methods

1. Anesthetize the mouse: inject intraperitoneally 10 ml/kg saline containing xylazine (1 mg/ml) and ketamine (5 mg/ml).

2. Check reflexes after 5 min (e.g., pinch footpad with forceps). If the mouse is in surgical tolerant anesthesia state, prepare for the surgery.

3. Place the mouse on the heated stage to prevent anesthesia-induced core temperature drop.

4. Apply eye protective cream to prevent cornea from drying out.

5. Disinfect the mouse belly with 0.02% chlorhexidine gluconate.

6. Use one pair of scissors to make 1 cm incision in the abdominal skin.

7. Use the second pair of scissors to make 1 cm incision in the muscular wall along the midline and gently stretch the small intestine (SI) (*see* **Note 1**).

8. Scan the SI by eye and identify PP structures.

9. Expose only small areas (1–2 cm long) at any time: once you locate a PP, partially close the skin incision with tissue glue (*see* **Note 2**).

10. Place a spring-loaded platform over the mouse and screw down until the cover glass makes contact with the PP.

11. Orient the PP according to the region you want to image.

12. Keep the PP almost immobilized against the mouse body using the platform and attached coverslip (*see* **Note 3**).

13. Use thermoconductive putty to surround the area around the PP and fill it with warm saline (*see* **Note 4**).

14. To further minimize the peristaltic movement, it is also possible to glue the tissue to the cover glass with tissue adhesive (*see* **Note 5**).

15. At least another system has been used to image PP and small intestine [11](*see* **Note 6**).

16. Measure the temperature at the interface between the PP and glass coverslip during and at the end of several imaging sessions using a dual temperature controller (*see* **Note 7**).

17. Maintain the anesthesia by intramuscular injections of 4 ml/kg of xylazine (1 mg/ml) and ketamine (5 mg/ml) every ~30 min. Always check reflexes 20–30 min after anesthesia. This step requires the interruption of the imaging process: different anesthetic options are available that allow continuous imaging (**steps 17** and **18**) (*see* **Note 8**).

18. For short-term intravital imaging (below 2 h), isoflurane at 2 % (v/v) can be used after the initial i.p. anesthesia induction (*see* **Note 9**).

19. For long-term intravital imaging, continuous i.p. injection of anesthetics (Ketamine 0.1 mg/ml, Xylazine 0.5 mg/ml, Fentanyl 5 μg/ml) using a syringe pump device with a flow rate of 0.2 ml/h in combination with isoflurane 0.5 Vol% (v/v) can be used.

20. Record time-lapse in 20–30 min block (*see* **Note 10**) for up to 3 h (*see* **Note 11**).

21. Save the data and analyze the movies (*see* **Note 12**).

4   Notes

1. Be careful not to damage any blood vessels while stretching the small intestine. An incision made further away from the diaphragm usually results in more stable images.

2. It is important not to close the skin too tightly: a herniated SI can undergo ischemia and infarction, affecting the immune process being imaged.

3. Avoid to push the cover glass too much into the PP, since it can damage the PP and alter the immune cell dynamics.

4. It is important to keep this area filled with saline at 37 °C to prevent dehydration and temperature drop.

5. To avoid blood vessels occlusion and necrosis, the adhesive has to be at least 2 mm from the site of imaging. For this reason, the SI surrounding the PP, but not PP itself, should be glued to the cover glass.

6. Other custom-made devices can be designed for this purpose: immobilization of the PP is crucial to generate usable time-lapse images.

7. The temperature needs to remain between 36 and 37 °C to avoid motility biases.

8. It is good practice to check on the condition of the mouse, as well as on the objective lens and on tissue immersion fluids lost from evaporation.

9. The use of isoflurane is possible only if the microscope room is properly ventilated.

10. Use the recorded time stamp if you want to concatenate movies acquired in different blocks. This is especially important to investigate cell dynamics longer than 20 min.

11. PP preparation is very delicate: damages can be induced during several steps of the procedure, including anesthesia,

surgery, and PP externalization. In addition, laser scanning can lead to both phototoxicity and photobleaching, especially if a high-intensity laser setting is used for a small area. For these reasons, it is safe to assume that the tissue begins to deteriorate 3 h from the starting of the procedure.

12. Analysis of a single two-photon movie can be extremely long, depending on the experimental settings and on the process under investigation: it can range from few hours for simple experiment up to several days for more complex experiments [12].

5   Choice of Fluorophore

The choice of fluorophore in 2P microscopy is critical for obtaining clear and trackable images: it is now common to use three or four fluorophores simultaneously (Table 1). However, complications can arise due to the intrinsic physical properties of the different fluorophores. A common problem is the inefficient excitation of all the fluorophores with a single wavelength. In our experience, excitation in the range of 850–900 nm is a good compromise for a broad range of fluorescent proteins, but the optimal excitation wavelength for the fluorophores of interest needs to be tailored to the specific experiment. As a general rule, it is wise to start testing the optimal excitation wavelength for each single fluorophore before moving to more complex settings. In addition, the density of a given fluorophore might compensate a non-optimal wavelength of excitation.

Another common problem is the emission spectral overlap, i.e., the fluorescence emitted from one fluorophore is also detected in the channel for a different fluorophore. This phenomenon can be corrected by the use of wavelength-specific dichroic mirrors and bandpass filters. However, dichroic mirrors and bandpass filters also lead to decreased brightness of the signal, and sometimes compromises need to be made between overlapping fluorescence and fluorescent intensity.

6   Strategies for Labeling Cells

The ability of tracking individual cells during intravital imaging is the direct result of target cell density: the optimal proportion between target and surrounding cells depends on the overall goal of the investigators. As a general rule, 0.1–1% of the total cells should be represented by the cells of interest [13]. However, for PP imaging, it can be useful to have additional fluorescent populations to define the PP micro-anatomy and the localization of the cells of interest. Based on the cells and the immune dynamics of interest, several strategies can be employed to achieve the perfect proportion of target and surrounding cells.

6.1 Short-term Adoptive Transfer

In PPs, ex vivo labeling of purified cells can be used for imaging T cells, B cells or other cell types that routinely recirculate in lymphoid organs. Intravenous injection of 10–50 millions of cell stained with vital dyes (CFSE or CellTraceViolet, for example) 6–24 h before imaging provides a cheap and quick strategy to achieve the desired cell density before two-photon imaging [14]. Since the dye intensity will decrease over time and will also be diluted with cell proliferation, ex vivo labeling can be used only for short-term imaging (i.e., entry and egress) or to highlight IFR or B follicle (Table 2).

6.2 Long-term Adoptive Transfer

For long-term imaging of immune dynamics of T cells and B cells in PPs, such as response to oral antigen or microbiome, fluorescent dyes cannot be used due to their half-life, but an ex vivo adoptive transfer can still be adopted. Mouse lines exist that express fluorescent proteins that ubiquitously label cells (Ubiquitin promoter-driven GFP or Actin promoter-driven CFP or RFP), and they can be used as a source of labeled recirculating cells for long-term PP imaging. In addition, mouse lines can also express fluorescent protein under a cell specific promoter, and at least one T cell-specific promoter-driven fluorescent reporter line exists (hCD2-DsRed in T cells [15]) (Table 2).

6.3 Reporter-Based Strategies

Cell populations characterized by slow/fast turnover (i.e., macrophages, DC, neutrophils) cannot reliably be transferred i.v. and imaged, due to poor tissue migration and/or survival. However, two strategies, based on in vivo frequency, are available to image such cells, assuming specific reporter line(s) could be used.

If the fluorescent protein expressing cells are less than 1% of total cells in the area of interest, reporter mice can be used directly for imaging, often in combination with adoptively transferred B cell or T cell to highlight PP micro-anatomy.

In this regard, mouse line expressing fluorescent protein under lineage promoter are useful for PP imaging (CD11c-YFP in dendritic cells, LysM-GFP in phagocytic cells such as macrophages [16] and neutrophils [17], Blimp1-YFP in plasma cells [18]) (Table 2).

Alternatively, if fluorescent cells of interest are present at high density but are anatomically restricted in a specific niche of PPs, bone marrow chimeras generated by mixing bone marrow from the chosen reporter mouse with bone marrow from a wild-type mouse can be used to achieve the desired density of fluorescent cells (Fig. 1 and Table 3).

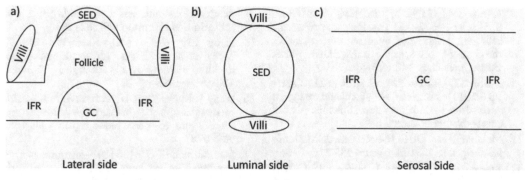

Fig. 1 Peyers' patches orientation for imaging different cell population. (**a**) Lateral view: this view is ideal to observe all the micro-anatomical niches. (**b**) Luminal view: this view is ideal for imaging processes in villi and SED, such as antigen entry and DC interaction in SED. (**c**) Serosal view: this view is ideal for imaging processes in germinal center and IFR, specially Tfh dynamics

6.4   Cre-/Lox-Based Strategies

When mice expressing the recombinase Cre under the control of a lineage-specific promoter are bred to mice with floxed stop codon in front of a fluorescent protein, the progeny can be a useful tool for PP imaging (Fig. 1 and Table 3). For example mice carrying both Cre recombinase driven by the endogenous Aicda locus and the reporter Rosa26lox-stop-lox-td Tomato have been recently used to image germinal centers [19]. In addition, the recombinase Cre can be introduced in cells through retroviral or lentiviral transduction [20] before adoptive transfer and/or bone marrow chimera.

Second-harmonic generation signal arise from organs rich in collagen and it is a label-free method of imaging structures like lymph node capsule.

Similarly, in PP, second-harmonic can be useful when imaging from the serosal or the luminal side.

References

1. Yamanaka T et al (2003) Microbial colonization drives lymphocyte accumulation and differentiation in the follicle-associated epithelium of Peyer's patches. J Immunol 170:816–822

2. Okada T et al (2002) Chemokine requirements for B cell entry to lymph nodes and Peyer's patches. J Exp Med 196:65–75

3. Schmidt TH, Bannard O, Gray EE, Cyster JG (2013) CXCR4 promotes B cell egress from Peyer's patches. J Exp Med 210:1099–1107

4. Reboldi A et al (2016) IgA production requires B cell interaction with subepithelial dendritic cells in Peyer's patches. Science 352: aaf4822–aaf4822

5. Rodda LB, Bannard O, Ludewig B, Nagasawa T, Cyster JG (2015) Phenotypic and morphological properties of germinal center dark zone Cxcl12-expressing reticular cells. J Immunol 195:4781–4791

6. Bergqvist P et al (2012) Re-utilization of germinal centers in multiple Peyer's patches results in highly synchronized, oligoclonal, and affinity-matured gut IgA responses. Mucosal Immunol 6:122–135

7. Gohda M, Kunisawa J, Miura F (2008) Sphingosine 1-phosphate regulates the egress of IgA plasmablasts from Peyer's patches for intestinal IgA responses. J Immunol 180:5335–5343. https://doi.org/10.1096/fj.14-251611

8. Lelouard H, Fallet M, de Bovis B, Méresse S, Gorvel J-P (2012) Peyer's patch dendritic cells sample antigens by extending dendrites through M cell-specific transcellular pores. Gastroenterology 142:592–601.e3

9. Arnon TI, Horton RM, Grigorova IL, Cyster JG (2013) Visualization of splenic marginal zone B-cell shuttling and follicular B-cell egress. Nature 493:684–688

10. McDole JR et al (2012) Goblet cells deliver luminal antigen to CD103. Nature 483:345–349

11. Kolesnikov M, Farache J, Shakhar G (2015) Intravital two-photon imaging of the gastrointestinal tract. J Immunol Methods 421:73–80. https://doi.org/10.1016/j.jim.2015.03.008

12. Beltman JB, Marée AFM, de Boer RJ (2009) Analysing immune cell migration. Nat Rev Immunol 9:789–798

13. Allen CDC, Okada T, Tang HL, Cyster JG (2007) Imaging of germinal center selection events during affinity maturation. Science 315:528–531

14. Henrickson SE et al (2008) T cell sensing of antigen dose governs interactive behavior with dendritic cells and sets a threshold for T cell activation. Nat Immunol 9:282–291

15. Kirby AC, Coles MC, Kaye PM (2009) Alveolar macrophages transport pathogens to lung draining lymph nodes. J Immunol 183:1983–1989

16. Wang J, Kubes P (2016) A reservoir of mature cavity macrophages that can rapidly invade visceral organs to affect tissue repair. Cell 165:668–678

17. Lämmermann T et al (2013) Neutrophil swarms require LTB4 and integrins at sites of cell death in vivo. Nature 498:371–375. https://doi.org/10.1038/nature12175

18. Fooksman DR et al (2010) Development and migration of plasma cells in the mouse lymph node. Immunity 33:118–127. https://doi.org/10.1016/j.immuni.2010.06.015

19. Tas JMJ et al (2016) Visualizing antibody affinity maturation in germinal centers. Science 351:1048–1054

20. Azar GA, Lemaitre F, Robey EA, Bousso P (2010) Subcellular dynamics of T cell immunological synapses and kinapses in lymph nodes. Proc Natl Acad Sci U S A 107:3675–3680

Chapter 11

Intravital Imaging of T Cells Within the Spinal Cord

Naoto Kawakami

Abstract

Intravital imaging is a powerful tool for analyzing cellular functions in living animals. In particular, after the two-photon microscopy technique was introduced, a number of studies have visualized important processes. Here, we describe the methods for performing intravital imaging of the central nervous system. This method can be used for imaging not only lymphocytes but also blood vessels for ischemia studies, as well as glia cell activities.

Key words Two-photon microscopy, Intravital imaging, Autoimmunity, Central nervous system, T cells

1 Introduction

The central nervous system (CNS) is known as an immune-privileged organ since it does not reject implants [1]. However, this characteristic does not mean that the CNS is completely isolated from the peripheral immune system. Although the CNS is separated via the blood–brain barrier (BBB), some T cells can penetrate into the CNS by passing through the BBB [2]. T cell infiltration becomes more obvious during inflammation in the CNS, which is observed in experimental autoimmune encephalomyelitis (EAE), an animal model of the human autoimmune disease multiple sclerosis (MS). By using conventional analysis of cell surface markers, it has been demonstrated that CNS-antigen-specific encephalitogenic T cells infiltrate into the CNS [3] and become activated there [4, 5]. Recently, our group used intravital imaging by two-photon microscopy and visualized the infiltration of encephalitogenic T cells into the CNS [2] as well as T cell activation in vivo [6, 7].

Intravital imaging by two-photon microscopy was initially used for imaging glia cells in the brain [8]. Later, the technique was introduced in immunological studies to track immune cells in organs. At first, imaging was performed in explanted peripheral

Masaru Ishii (ed.), *Intravital Imaging of Dynamic Bone and Immune Systems: Methods and Protocols*, Methods in Molecular Biology, vol. 1763, https://doi.org/10.1007/978-1-4939-7762-8_11, © Springer Science+Business Media, LLC 2018

lymph nodes [9, 10] and soon followed by imaging of lymph nodes in vivo [11]. Since then, this method has become suitable for imaging cells in live animals at single cell resolution for extended time periods and has been used for many studies [12]. Early stages of two-photon intravital imaging were mainly used to detect parameters of cellular movement, including motility, the motility coefficient, and the meandering index. Recently by using functional florescent proteins, cellular functions, such as changes in intracellular calcium [7] and activation [6, 13, 14], can be monitored in real time.

There are, in general, several critical factors for successful intravital imaging. One of the most important factors is the proper labeling of the target cells. Currently, there are many transgenic mouse lines that express fluorescent proteins in specific cell lineages [15]. Most of these transgenic lines express sufficient amounts of fluorescent proteins and can be used for intravital imaging; however, in a few of them, the expression level is too low for signal detection. Additionally, researchers need to consider specific future of some organs. For example, CNS contains myelin, which scatters both excitation and emission light, making the signal weaker. Spleen is filled with red blood cells which efficiently absorb excitation light. Another factor is the stabilization of the target tissue. This stabilization is relatively easier for CNS tissues since they are surrounded by hard bones. CNS tissues can be stabilized by mechanical fixation. However, too much stress can disturb blood flow or destroy the tissue.

We usually use retroviral gene transfer to label T cells. The detailed method has been previously described for rat T cells [3] and mouse T cells [7]. Retroviral gene transfer can be used for any type of proliferating cell. To label the nonproliferating cells, lentiviruses need to be used. In general, the signals from retrovirally labeled cells are weaker than chemically labeled cells but sufficient for intravital imaging. Alternatively, chemical dyes such as 5-(and 6)-carboxyfluorescein diacetate succinimidyl ester (CFSE) [16] or cells prepared from transgenic animals can be used [15].

2 Materials

2.1 Machines

Two-photon microscope.

Surgical microscope.

Ventilator for small animals (Inspira or equivalent one).

Isoflurane vaporizer.

Gas monitor (Dräger PM8050 or equivalent one).

Hair shaver.

Dental drill.

Tissue chopper.

2.2   Instruments

Vein catheter (26 G).

Intubation tube (14 G or 16 G).

Fine forceps.

Spring scissors.

Surgical knives.

Slice anchor.

2.3   Buffers

HBSS (10×) (Prepare 1× solution before use by adding 1 g/l $NaHCO_3$).

NaCl	80 g/l
KCl	4 g/l
KH_2PO_4	0.6 g/l
Glucose	10 g/l
Na_2HPO_4	0.478 g/l

2.4   Others

Carbogen gas.

Oxygen gas.

1.5% low melting temperature agarose in PBS.

3   Methods

3.1   Presurgery Treatment

1. Anesthetize the animal (*see* **Note 1**).

2. Insert a catheter into the tail vein. After connecting a three-way stop cock, stabilize with plaster (*see* **Note 2**).

3. Insert an intubation tube into the trachea (*see* **Note 3**). Fix the inserted intubation tube by using superglue.

4. Connect the intubation tube with an animal ventilator (*see* **Note 4**). Start supplying a mixture of oxygen and room air with anesthesia gas (*see* **Note 5**). The schematic representation of the gas line is illustrated in Fig. 1.

5. Maintain the body temperature at 37 °C by heating (*see* **Note 6**).

6. Put Vaseline on both eyes to prevent drying.

3.2   Surgery to Prepare Spinal Cord Window

In this part of the protocol, a spinal cord window is prepared at the lumbar spinal cord since encephalitogenic T cells begin infiltrating there [17]. In addition, this is the part where the spinal cord is most superficial and easy to access. Typically, the spinal cord window is prepared at level L1.

1. Shave the hair around the imaging area by using a hair shaver.

2. Make a 1–1.5 cm cut on the skin using a surgical knife.

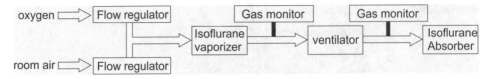

Fig. 1 The schematic representation of the gas line

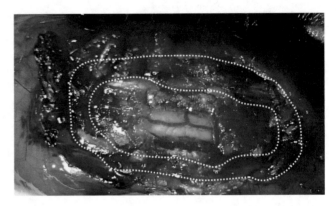

Fig. 2 Spinal cord window surrounded by agarose ring. Agarose ring is outlined with dotted line

3. Stabilize the spinal cord (*see* **Note 7**).

4. Remove muscles on the spinal cord using the surgical knife (*see* **Note 8**).

5. Using a dental drill, perforate both sides of the vertebra (*see* **Notes 9** and **10**).

6. Remove the dura mater using fine forceps if it is necessary (*see* **Note 11**).

7. Make an agarose ring around the imaging window (*see* **Note 12**) (Fig. 2).

8. Start intravital imaging.

3.3 Imaging of Spinal Cord Explants

Since the penetration depth of the two-photon microscope is limited, it is hard to image deep inside the spinal cord, parenchyma. Using an endoscope, it is possible to perform imaging in the CNS parenchyma [18]. Since the endoscope must be inserted precisely into the target location, this method requires intensive training and gives limited view of imaging. An alternative method of explant imaging of the spinal cord, which is easier to perform but less physiological, is described in this section.

1. Dissect the spinal cord from the animal (*see* **Note 13**).

2. Make acute slices (thickness: 300 μm) using a tissue chopper (*see* **Note 14**).

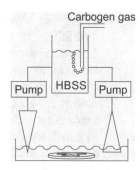

Fig. 3 The schematic representation of buffer circulation system for imaging in the explants

3. Store the acute slices in ice-cold HBSS bubbled with carbogen gas.

4. Put a slice into the imaging chamber and stabilize with a slice anchor (*see* **Note 15**).

5. Start the buffer circulation system (*see* **Note 16**) (Fig. 3).

3.4 Image Acquisition

1. Find the region of interest (*see* **Note 17**).

2. Select the z-volume (*see* **Note 18**).

3. Set the z-interval (*see* **Note 19**).

4. Set the time interval (*see* **Note 20**).

5. Set averaging (*see* **Notes 21** and **22**).

3.5 Image Analysis

Cellular motility is one of the most commonly analyzed parameters. Values can be obtained from coordinate information from each cell at each time point. Using the pixel size and time interval, cellular motility can be calculated. We use the manual tracking plugin in Fiji to perform the analysis. Alternatively, the automatic tracking function in a commercial software such as Imaris could be another option.

4 Notes

1. At first, the animals are kept in a chamber supplied with 4% isoflurane. Then, a mixture of fentanyl-based anesthesia is injected. For rats, a mixture of 5 µg/kg fentanyl, 2 mg/kg midazolam, and 150 µg/kg medetomidine is injected intramuscularly. For mice, a mixture of 50 µg/kg fentanyl, 50 µg/kg midazolam, and 500 µg/kg medetomidine is injected intraperitoneally. Other anesthesia reagents can be used. IMPORTANT: keep contact with local authorities to use anesthetics.

2. Wash the blood remains in the catheter and 3-way cock carefully with sterile PBS or saline, which may otherwise clot. It is recommended to flow physiological buffer during intravital imaging to avoid dehydration of the animal and prevent clotting in the catheter. This cannulation protocol is used mainly for rats. For mice, it is better to cannulate the jugular vein. Alternatively, 30 G needles attached to tubes can be inserted into the mouse tail vein. The vein catheter is not absolutely necessary, but it can be useful for intravenous injections during intravital imaging since blood vessels tend to shrink in anesthetized animals.

3. After disinfection of the skin with 70% ethanol, cut the skin, and expose the salivary glands. Using forceps, carefully move both salivary glands, and expose the trachea located between the salivary glands. The trachea is covered with a thin layer of muscles that can be removed by forceps. Using spring scissors, cut a part of the trachea, and carefully insert the intubation tube. Intubation tubes can be inserted into the trachea but not into the primary bronchus. The intubation tube must be thick enough so as not to have any space between the tube and the trachea.

4. The volume and frequency of ventilation must be decided by the size of the animal [19].

5. Isoflurane (1.5% for rats and 1.0% for mice) is used in our lab. The concentrations of O_2 and CO_2 in the inspiratory and expiratory air are continuously monitored. Typically, 50–60% of O_2 in the inspiratory air is used to provide sufficient oxygen saturation in the animal, which is also monitored.

6. Monitor body temperature in the rectum by inserting a small probe. It is desirable to use a heating function connected with the temperature measurement.

7. We use a custom-made fixation device, which is shaped like forceps. Using a pair of this device, both upper and lower parts of the spinal cord are clamped and stabilized. A similar device is illustrated in [20]. We also use commercially available devices, for example, STS-A for mice and STS-B for rats (both from Narishige).

8. Remove as much muscle as possible from the imaging window. Any remaining muscle may contain blood vessels that can induce continuous blood contamination into the imaging window. Since red blood cells efficiently absorb infrared laser, it is hard to acquire images if blood is present in the imaging window. This process should be done under a surgical microscope, which provides a better view of the muscles.

9. It is recommended to use a drill that produces less vibrations. When the vertebra is pushed by the drill and attached directly to the spinal cord, vibrations can be transferred to the spinal cord and cause damages, which may mislead the experimental results. This situation needs to be considered more when the spinal cord is inflamed since the spinal cord is often swollen. One way to control the possible damage would be to image between vertebrae without opening. Alternatively, bone rongeurs can be used to remove bone. With this instrument, there is no danger of producing vibrations. For the mouse spinal cord, the vertebrae are thin enough to be cut by scissors. In this case, spring scissors with angled blades are a better choice. In any case, pay attention to not touch the spinal cord.

10. Typically, opening one vertebra provides a sufficient imaging area. If a larger imaging area is needed, more vertebrae can be removed, which may reduce the stability of the image due to reduced rigidity.

11. The imaging condition is more similar to the physiological condition with dura mater. On the other hand, since the dura mater is a relatively dense structure, it reduces the quality of images of the spinal cord pia mater and parenchyma.

12. It is recommended to use low melting temperature agarose with concentrations of 1–2% in PBS at 37 °C. Prepare a ring structure around the imaging window. This ring is necessary to keep the buffer between the spinal cord and the objective lens since objective lens with long working distance is often used. If other type of objective lens is used, this step may not be necessary. To avoid damage induced by heat, pay attention to the temperature of agarose, and do not apply the molten agarose directly onto the imaging window.

13. The spinal cord should be free of damage. Otherwise, it becomes difficult to prepare acute slices in the next step.

14. The thickness of the tissue slice can be changed although it is hard to make the slices thinner than 300 µm. Instead of using a tissue chopper, a vibratome can be used. In this case, the spinal cord should be embedded in low melting temperature agarose before cutting.

15. The thickness of the slice anchor must be same to the thickness of the acute slice. Otherwise, the slice will be pressed too strongly, and its shape will continuously change during imaging or slice moves according to buffer flow. When inverted microscopy is used, a glass bottom plate should be used for better image quality.

16. It is critical to keep temperature around the acute slice at 35–37 °C. This can be done either using chamber or warming buffer in water bath.

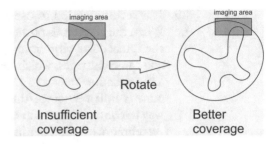

Fig. 4 The schematic view of imaging area on curved spinal cord

Insufficient coverage

Rotate

Better coverage

17. The surface of the spinal cord is not flat but curved, which means that the z-position of the surface of the spinal cord differs even within a single image. To avoid this, the top of the spinal cord is usually the best place for imaging, but this is a place where major vessels are located and is not too interesting. In this case, rotate the animal, and obtain a better position. (Fig. 4).

18. In our experimental setup with retrovirally transduced GFP-expressing rat T cells in the spinal cord with dura mater, the maximum penetration depth is approximately 200 μm.

19. The z-interval must be decided based on the target cells. Typically, lymphocytes have diameters of up to 10 μm. If a z-interval of more than 5 μm is used, the cell is detected only once, and this may result in unclear cellular images. In addition, to detect subcellular structures, for example, to detect the intracellular location of NFAT-GFP [6, 13], a more precise z-interval is necessary.

20. It is important to keep the time interval constant to compare cellular motility between different movies. Additionally, the time interval must be short enough to be able to track a single cell among many cells. Typically, time intervals of 30 s to 1 min are used to track moving lymphocytes in the organs.

21. To improve the image quality, multiple averaging is recommended. For detecting very fast events or cellular motility, line averaging is better. If not, frame averaging might reduce phototoxicity.

22. All parameters between **Notes 14** and **17** influence the quality of images. In general, a longer time is needed to obtain higher quality images. One must find a balance between image quality and time.

Acknowledgements

This work was supported by DFG (Transregio 128, Heisenberg fellowship and individual grant KA2951/2-1), the Novartis Foundation for Therapeutic Research, Max-Planck Society, and LMU Munich.

References

1. Engelhardt B, Vajkoczy P, Weller RO (2017) The movers and shapers in immune privilege of the CNS. Nat Immunol 18(2):123–131

2. Bartholomäus I et al (2009) Effector T cell interactions with meningeal vascular structures in nascent autoimmune CNS lesions. Nature 462:94–98

3. Flügel A et al (1999) Gene transfer into CD4 + T lymphocytes: Green fluorescent protein engineered, encephalitogenic T cells used to illuminate immune responses in the brain. Nat Med 5(7):843–847

4. Flügel A et al (2001) Migratory activity and functional changes of green fluorescent effector T cells before and during experimental autoimmune encephalomyelitis. Immunity 14(5):547–560

5. Kawakami N et al (2004) The activation status of neuroantigen-specific T cells in the target organ determines the clinical outcome of autoimmune encephalomyelitis. J Exp Med 199(2):185–197

6. Pesic M et al (2013) 2-photon imaging of phagocyte-mediated T cell activation in the CNS. J Clin Invest 123(3):1192–1201

7. Mues M et al (2013) Real-time in vivo analysis of T cell activation in the central nervous system using a genetically encoded calcium indicator. Nat Med 19(6):778–783

8. Denk W, Strickler JH, Webb WW (1990) 2-Photon laser scanning fluorescence microscopy. Science 248:73–76

9. Stoll S et al (2002) Dynamic imaging of T cell-dendritic cell interactions in lymph nodes. Science 296:1873–1876

10. Miller MJ et al (2002) Two-photon imaging of lymphocyte motility and antigen response in intact lymph node. Science 296:1869–1873

11. Cahalan MD et al (2003) Real-time imaging of lymphocytes in vivo. Curr Opin Immunol 15(4):372–377

12. Benechet AP, Menon M, Khanna KM (2014) Visualizing T cell migration in situ. Front Immunol 5:363

13. Lodygin D et al (2013) A combination of fluorescent NFAT and H2B sensors uncovers dynamics of T cell activation in real time during CNS autoimmunity. Nat Med 19(6):784–790

14. Komatsu N et al (2011) Development of an optimized backbone of FRET biosensors for kinases and GTPases. Mol Biol Cell 22(23):4647–4656

15. Kawakami N (2016) In vivo imaging in autoimmune diseases in the central nervous system. Allergol Int 65(3):235–242

16. Gerard A et al (2014) Detection of rare antigen-presenting cells through T cell-intrinsic meandering motility, mediated by Myo1g. Cell 158(3):492–505

17. Arima Y et al (2012) Regional neural activation defines a gateway for autoreactive T cells to cross the bood-brain barrier. Cell 148(3):447

18. Barretto RPJ et al (2011) Time-lapse imaging of disease progression in deep brain areas using fluorescence microendoscopy. Nat Med 17(2):223–228

19. Stahl WR (1967) Scaling of respiratory variables in mammals. J Appl Physiol 22(3):453–460

20. Davalos D et al (2008) Stable in vivo imaging of densely populated glia, axons and blood vessels in the mouse spinal cord using two-photon microscopy. J Neurosci Methods 169(1):1–7

Chapter 12

Kidney Imaging: Intravital Microscopy

Takashi Hato, Seth Winfree, and Pierre C. Dagher

Abstract

Intravital two-photon microscopy is a powerful imaging tool for investigating various biological processes in live animals. This chapter describes an overview of intravital imaging of the rodent kidney including animal surgery, characteristics of renal tubular autofluorescence, in vivo use of fluorescent probes, and renal immune-cell tracking.

Key words Kidney, Intravital two-photon microscopy, Oxidative stress, Renal immune cell imaging

1 Introduction

The kidney is a highly complex organ consisting of a large set of diverse cell types organized to form an intricate network of three-dimensional structures. Various microscopy-based imaging modalities have been the cornerstone of kidney research and helped unravel some of the complex spatiotemporal biological phenomena occurring in this organ. However, the recent advances in imaging techniques such as intravital two-photon microscopy, super-resolution microscopy and tissue clearing methods, offer immense additional potential to move past the status quo [1, 2]. Intravital two-photon microscopy was first applied to the live kidney in 2002 and since then this technique has been widely adopted with successful attempt to investigate various biological questions [3–7]. While the imaging depth remains a challenge (~100 μm from the surface), intravital two-photon microscopy enables the real-time visualization and quantification of objects and events at subcellular levels—a major strength that is not achievable by other tools. In this chapter, we describe our two-photon microscopy protocols as applied to specific questions in kidney research. We first describe our approach to identify renal tubular subsegments based on their autofluorescence characteristics. We next show representative in vivo applications of fluorescent probes to evaluate biological properties of interest such

Masaru Ishii (ed.), *Intravital Imaging of Dynamic Bone and Immune Systems: Methods and Protocols*, Methods in Molecular Biology, vol. 1763, https://doi.org/10.1007/978-1-4939-7762-8_12, © Springer Science+Business Media, LLC 2018

as endotoxin uptake and its effect on oxidative stress and mitochondrial membrane potential. Finally, we describe spatiotemporal renal immune cell imaging and its data processing.

2   Materials

2.1   Microscopy

Olympus FV1000-MPE confocal/multiphoton microscope equipped with a Spectra Physics MaiTai Deep See laser and external gallium arsenide 12-bit detectors. The system is mounted on an Olympus Ix81 inverted microscope stand with a Nikon 20× and 70× NA 1.2 water-immersion objective.

2.2   Reagents

1. FITC-inulin (Sigma-Aldrich).

2. Tetramethylrhodamine methyl ester (TMRM, a mitochondrial membrane potential indicator).

3. Oxidative stress probes. Carboxy-2′,7′-dichlorodihydrofluorescein diacetate (H_2DCFDA) and dihydroethydium.

4. Labeled-lipopolysaccharide (LPS). Alexa-594 LPS (LPS from E coli 055:B5). Alternatively, conjugate Alexa hydrazide to LPS (*S. minnesota* Re 595) using established protocols [8]. The conjugate is separated from free probe using PD-10 columns.

5. High molecular weight poly (I:C) rhodamine (a fluorescently labeled ligand of toll-like receptor 3).

6. Hoechst 33342 (nuclear staining).

2.3   Surgical Instruments

1. Catheter (polyethylene tubing, PE50; BD).

2. 4.0 nonabsorbable silk suture.

3. Isoflurane, anesthesia circuit, warming pad.

4. Glass bottom culture dish (50/40 mm, Glass thick 0.17 mm/#1.5).

3   Methods

3.1   Animal Surgery

Anesthetize with an isoflurane/O_2 mixture (3% for induction and 1% or less for maintenance of anesthesia). An induction chamber is used for induction and an anesthesia circuit is used during surgery and imaging. The animal is placed on a thermostatically controlled warming pad. A rectal probe is used to monitor temperature. Expose the jugular vein and insert a PE50 catheter under a dissecting microscope (Fig. 1a). Expose the kidney via a 1.5 cm flank incision and loosely suture the skin to stabilize the kidney exposure. Transport the animal to a microscopic stage and place the kidney in a coverslip-bottomed cell culture dish filled with normal saline (Fig. 1b).

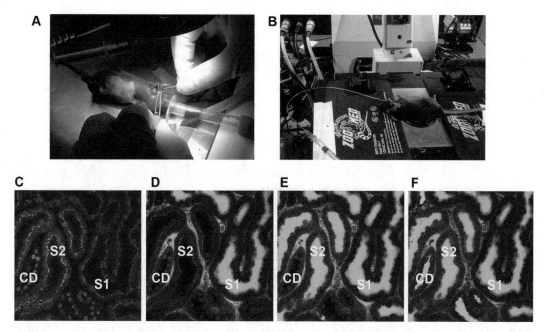

Fig. 1 (**a**) Animal preparation for intravital kidney imaging. A PE50 catheter is inserted in the right jugular vein under a dissection microscope. The left flank is shaved for kidney exposure. (**b**) The animal is placed on an inverted Olympus FV1000-MPE confocal/multiphoton microscope. The left kidney is exposed and placed in a glass bottom culture dish that contains a rubber pad to stabilize the kidney. A catheter and rectal thermometer are in place. (**b**) A representative mouse renal cortex (C57BL/6) imaged with two-photon microscopy. Hoechst (blue) stained nuclei and is brightest in the collecting duct. The green and red represent autofluorescence. S2 proximal tubules have bright green pigments in the apical cytosolic space whereas S1 proximal tubules have dark brown pigments. The S2 cytosolic green autofluorescence is brighter than that of S1. Distal segments exhibit very weak green autofluorescence. The absolute appearance of autofluorescence can vary depending on microscope setup (laser wavelength, laser power, detector sensitivity) and other factors (animal strains, disease condition, and concomitant use of fluorescent probes). (**d–f**) The anatomical sequence of S1 and S2 is confirmed by FITC-inulin infusion. FITC-inulin was injected and images were obtained every 1 s. Figures **c** and **d** reproduced from Kalakeche et al. 2011 with permission from Journal of the American Society of Nephrology [11]

3.2 Identification of Kidney Tubular Subsegments Based on Autofluorescence Signatures

Images are acquired with an Olympus FV1000-MPE confocal/multiphoton microscope. The laser is tuned to 800-nm excitation. To obtain reproducible, quantitative images, careful attention must be paid to image acquisition parameters including laser power, photomultiplier tube (PMT) detector gain, and the black level of the PMT amplifier (offset) [9]. Our typical setup is laser power 15%, green PMT voltage 750 with offset 45%, and red PMT 575 with offset 35%.

The dominant structures seen in the renal cortex are S1 and S2 proximal tubules as well as some distal segments like collecting ducts. S1 and S2 subsegments can be distinguished by their unique autofluorescence signatures (*see* **Note 1**). S1 tubules have brown-colored punctate pigments beneath the brush border. In contrast, S2 tubules have green punctate pigments (Fig. 1c). In addition, the S2 cytosolic green signal is slightly brighter than that of S1. The distal segments have minimal autofluorescence. Superficial glomeruli are rare [10] and they do not exhibit autofluorescence.

The S1, S2 autofluorescence signatures may appear different when the kidney is diseased or is imaged with bright fluorescent dyes. Different strains or species would also have a different auto-fluorescence pattern. To confirm the anatomical sequence of S1 (upstream) and S2 (downstream), one can inject fluorescently tagged inulin intravenously (25 ng/kg) and obtain a time-series (Fig. 1d–f). The urine flow is sufficiently slow to distinguish S1, S2, and distal segments.

3.3 Application of Fluorescent Probes in Live Animals

3.3.1 Fluorescently Labeled LPS

To study the uptake of LPS by proximal tubules [11], resuspend Alexa-568 LPS in normal saline and inject intraperitoneally (100 μg in 100 μL normal saline for a 20 g mouse; 5 mg/kg) and obtain images 4 h later (Fig. 2a).

3.3.2 TMRM

Prepare a stock solution (2.5 μg/μL; 5 mg TMRM in 2 mL DMSO). For a 20 g mouse, take 10 μL (25 μg) from the stock and dilute in 5 mL normal saline. Inject 50 μL (0.25 μg) intravenously and image 20 min later (Fig. 2b; *see* **Note 2**).

3.3.3 Carboxy-H₂DCFDA

Dissolve 5 mg H_2DCFDA in 200 μL ethanol and divide into 30 μL (750 μg) per tube aliquots. Wrap the stock solutions in aluminum foil and store them in −80° freezer. Immediately before use, dilute the 30 μL stock with 500 μL PBS (room temperature) and inject 100 μL (150 μg) intravenously (7.5 mg/kg for a 20 g mouse). Obtain images 20 min later (Fig. 2c). Minimize exposure of H_2DCFDA to ambient light or microscope arc lamp in order to avoid nonspecific excitement of the dye (*see* **Note 3**).

3.3.4 Dihydroethidium

Prepare stock solutions (2 mg/mL in DMSO). Take 30 μL (60 μg) from the stock and redilute in normal saline and administer intravenously (3 mg/kg for a 20 g mouse). Obtain images 60 min later (Fig. 2d; *see* **Note 4**).

3.3.5 Hoechst

Dilute the stock solution (10 mg/mL) 1:10 and inject 50 μL (50 μg/50 μL) intraperitoneally 1 h before imaging.

3.4 Imaging Renal Immune Cells

Intravital two-photon microscopy has an enormous advantage for studying immune-cell trafficking with great temporal and spatial resolution [12]. The key to success is to stabilize the animal and kidney on the microscope stage for long time. Careful consideration should be given to upright versus inverted microscopy. An additional supporting device such as a kidney cup may be required [13]. Renal immune cells exhibit very weak autofluorescence compared to the renal tubules. Therefore, fluorescent labeling is necessary for imaging.

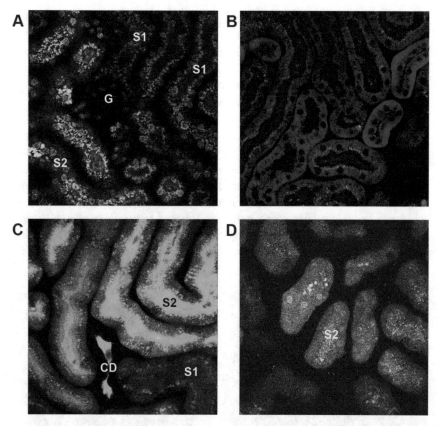

Fig. 2 (**a**) A representative image of LPS uptake by S1 proximal tubules. Alexa-labeled LPS (red) was administered intraperitoneally 4 h before imaging. Superficial glomeruli are rare but can be imaged as shown. Nuclei (blue) were stained with Hoechst. (**b**) A mitochondrial membrane potential maker, TMRM (red), was administered intravenously 20 min before imaging. (**c**) An oxidative stress marker, carboxy-H$_2$DCFDA (green), was administered intravenously 20 min before imaging. The animal was injected with unlabeled LPS 4 h before carboxy-H$_2$DCFDA administration. Note the prominent oxidative stress in the S2 brush border that makes up the bulk of the S2 lumen. (**d**) An oxidative stress marker, dihydroethidium (red), is intercalated with nuclear DNA in the S2 tubule of LPS-treated mice

3.4.1 Time-series imaging

CX$_3$CR1-EGFP mouse, in which myeloid cells exhibit EGFP green fluorescence, is injected with 10 µg rhodamine-poly (I:C) (a ligand of toll-like receptor 3) (*see* **Note 5**). Images are obtained every 18 s for 1 h and 45 min and are reconstructed as a video using ImageJ (Fig. 3a–d; Supplemental Data 3 in ref. 14, reproduced from Hato et al., 2015 with permission from Journal of the American Society of Nephrology). This time interval is long enough to monitor the animal's condition between imaging yet short enough to capture the behavior of immune cells with sufficient detail. To minimize motion artifact, anesthesia dose is kept low (<1% isoflurane) and the kidney is placed in an imaging dish with a ring-shaped rubber pad.

3.4.2 Data Processing   Existing cell-tracking software/programs were unable to recognize poly (I:C) positive cells properly. This is because these cells comprise multiple punctate structures (red) with poor cell body delineation (Fig. 3a). We therefore developed a Custom Plugin "Trk_PP" for preprocessing of data sets. This plugin generates a center-of-mass image for cells with poor cell body delineation or punctate signatures [14]. The center-of-mass image is then used in the "TrackMate" plugin to generate tracks of cell movement in ImageJ. The source code is available as a Maven project at https:// github.com/icbm-iupui/track-processing. This plugin can be useful for cell-tracking analysis when the cells have various compartmentalized fluorescent signals.

"Trk_PP" installs in Fiji and ImageJ under the "Plugins" directory and "Tracking" subdirectory under "PreProcessing." "Trk_PP" generates three outputs: (1) the processed form of the original

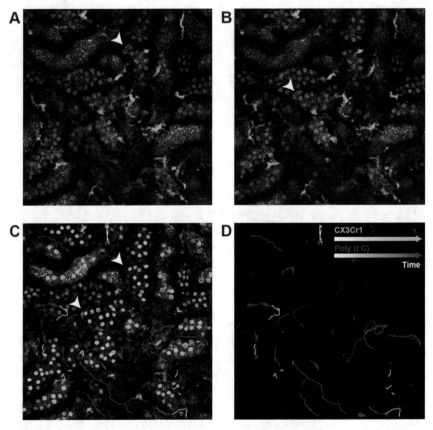

Fig. 3 (**a** and **b**) The CX3CR1-eGFP mouse (green) was injected with rhodamine-poly (I:C) (red). The animal was preconditioned with LPS that increased the number and activity of myeloid cells in the kidney. Nuclei were stained with Hoechst. Arrowhead followed a specific macrophage over time. (**c** and **d**) Traces represent the traveled path of mobile macrophages expressing CX_3CR1 (green) and rhodamine-poly (I:C) (red) over 1 h and 45 min. Color intensity of traces is graded as a function of time. Figures reproduced from Hato et al. 2015 with permission from Journal of the American Society of Nephrology [14]

data "Processed," (2) the mask image of the regions used to define the center-of-mass points "Mask of regions," and (3) an image containing the center-of-mass as a dot with a user selected diameter, "center-of-mass."

4   Notes

1. A number of endogenous metabolites possess fluorophore properties, known as autofluorescence [15]. While this intrinsic fluorescence property has been exploited to measure certain metabolites such as reduced forms of nicotinamide adenine dinucleotide, a comprehensive catalog of metabolites that contribute to autofluorescence in the kidney is not available.

2. TMRM is a cationic fluorescent dye that is sequestered by live mitochondria in proportion to their membrane potential. The heterogeneous distribution of TMRM may reflect "microcirculation failure" [5].

   The proper dose of fluorescent dye for intravital imaging is often unknown. We typically refer to in vitro data using an estimated blood volume of the animal as a starting point then titrate the dose as needed. Similarly, the way in which a fluorescent probe is taken up by live kidney is often unknown (i.e., basolateral versus filtered and taken up from the tubular lumen). A time-series imaging may be useful to determine the behavior of a dye of interest [16].

3. H_2DCFDA is sensitive to arc lamp light. Artifactual photooxidation of the dye occurs especially in the presence of LPS [14]. We do not recommend examining the tissue through the eyepiece once the dye is injected in order to minimize artificial excitement of the dye.

   In our model of LPS-induced kidney injury, oxidative stress is most notable in the S2 brush border. The concentrated dye in the collecting duct emits bright green fluorescence regardless of oxidation (Fig. 2c). We also note that carboxy-H_2DCFDA leaks out of the cell 30–60 min after injection even though it is engineered to delay the leak via cleavage of acetate and ester groups.

4. Dihydroethidium is a cell permeant fluorescent dye that detects cytosolic superoxide. Once the dye is oxidized, it intercalates with the cell's DNA and emits bright orange fluorescence from the nucleus.

5. Poly (I:C) uptake by myeloid cells is significantly increased with LPS preconditioning [14]. Wild-type non-preconditioned C57/BL6 mice have minimal poly (I:C) uptake.

Acknowledgements

This work was supported by National Institutes of Health (NIH) Grant R01 DK080067 (NIH), VA Merit (1I01BX002901-01A2), O'Brien Center grant P30DK079312 (NIH) to P.C.D. and Dialysis Clinics Inc. and Indiana Clinical and Translational Sciences Institute to T.H.

References

1. Torres R, Velazquez H, Chang JJ, Levene MJ, Moeckel G, Desir GV, Safirstein R (2016) Three-dimensional morphology by multiphoton microscopy with clearing in a model of cisplatin-induced CKD. J Am Soc Nephrol 27(4):1102–1112

2. Unnersjo-Jess D, Scott L, Blom H, Brismar H (2016) Super-resolution stimulated emission depletion imaging of slit diaphragm proteins in optically cleared kidney tissue. Kidney Int 89(1):243–247

3. Dunn KW, Sandoval RM, Kelly KJ, Dagher PC, Tanner GA, Atkinson SJ, Bacallao RL, Molitoris BA (2002) Functional studies of the kidney of living animals using multicolor two-photon microscopy. Am J Physiol Cell Physiol 283(3):C905–C916

4. Peti-Peterdi J, Kidokoro K, Riquier-Brison A (2015) Novel in vivo techniques to visualize kidney anatomy and function. Kidney Int 88(1):44–51

5. Nakano D, Doi K, Kitamura H, Kuwabara T, Mori K, Mukoyama M, Nishiyama A (2015) Reduction of tubular flow rate as a mechanism of oliguria in the early phase of endotoxemia revealed by intravital imaging. J Am Soc Nephrol 26(12):3035–3044

6. Oberbarnscheidt MH, Zeng Q, Li Q, Dai H, Williams AL, Shlomchik WD, Rothstein DM, Lakkis FG (2014) Non-self recognition by monocytes initiates allograft rejection. J Clin Invest 124(8):3579–3589

7. Hall AM, Crawford C, Unwin RJ, Duchen MR, Peppiatt-Wildman CM (2011) Multiphoton imaging of the functioning kidney. J Am Soc Nephrol 22(7):1297–1304

8. Triantafilou K, Triantafilou M, Fernandez N (2000) Lipopolysaccharide (LPS) labeled with Alexa 488 hydrazide as a novel probe for LPS binding studies. Cytometry 41(4):316–320

9. Sandoval RM, Wagner MC, Patel M, Campos-Bilderback SB, Rhodes GJ, Wang E, Wean SE, Clendenon SS, Molitoris BA (2012) Multiple factors influence glomerular albumin permeability in rats. J Am Soc Nephrol 23(3):447–457

10. Schiessl IM, Bardehle S, Castrop H (2013) Superficial nephrons in BALB/c and C57BL/6 mice facilitate in vivo multiphoton microscopy of the kidney. PLoS One 8(1):e52499

11. Kalakeche R, Hato T, Rhodes G, Dunn KW, El-Achkar TM, Plotkin Z, Sandoval RM, Dagher PC (2011) Endotoxin uptake by S1 proximal tubular segment causes oxidative stress in the downstream S2 segment. J Am Soc Nephrol 22(8):1505–1516

12. Phan TG, Bullen A (2010) Practical intravital two-photon microscopy for immunological research: faster, brighter, deeper. Immunol Cell Biol 88(4):438–444

13. Camirand G, Li Q, Demetris AJ, Watkins SC, Shlomchik WD, Rothstein DM, Lakkis FG (2011) Multiphoton intravital microscopy of the transplanted mouse kidney. Am J Transplant 11(10):2067–2074

14. Hato T, Winfree S, Kalakeche R, Dube S, Kumar R, Yoshimoto M, Plotkin Z, Dagher PC (2015) The macrophage mediates the renoprotective effects of endotoxin preconditioning. J Am Soc Nephrol 26(6):1347–1362

15. Berezin MY, Achilefu S (2010) Fluorescence lifetime measurements and biological imaging. Chem Rev 110(5):2641–2684

16. Hato T, Friedman AN, Mang HE, Plotkin Z, Dube S, Hutchins GD, Territo PR, McCarthy BP, Riley AA, Pichumani K, Malloy CR, Harris RA, Dagher PC, Sutton TA (2016) Novel application of complimentary imaging techniques to examine in vivo glucose metabolism in the kidney. Am J Physiol Renal Physiol 310:F717–F727

Chapter 13

Intravital Imaging of Liver Cell Dynamics

Sayaka Matsumoto, Junichi Kikuta, and Masaru Ishii

Abstract

The liver is a vital organ in the body. It has various essential functions, including detoxification, protein synthesis, and control of infection. Because of its medical importance, liver diseases such as hepatitis and cirrhosis can be crucial for an individual. Exploring dynamics of living cells in the liver would provide the clues for understanding the pathology. However, due to its technical difficulty, few studies have used intravital liver imaging. To resolve this, we have established a novel imaging system for visualizing liver cell dynamics in living animals.

Herein we describe the methodology for visualizing the in vivo behavior of liver cells using intravital multiphoton microscopy. This approach will be useful for understanding the pathogenesis of liver disorders, as well as liver biology, in vivo.

Key words Intravital imaging, Multiphoton microscopy, Hepatocyte, Liver sinusoidal endothelial cell, Kupffer cell

1 Introduction

The liver is the largest organ in the abdominal cavity and perfused by a great volume of blood [1]. Various types of cells exist around a network of capillaries called sinusoids: abundant hepatocytes, and specialized cells, such as liver sinusoidal endothelial cells (LSECs), Kupffer cells, and lymphocytes. This unique structure and cellular population allow the liver to serve many vital functions, including detoxification, protein synthesis, bile production, glucose metabolism, and control of infection.

Because it is difficult to visualize the inner liver tissue in living animals, only a few in vivo studies have described the mechanisms of liver diseases. Although the cell population, morphology, and structure in liver tissues can be analyzed by conventional methods such as histological analysis and flow cytometry, these methods only allow for the evaluation of cell shape and molecular expression, but cannot observe the movement and interaction of different cell types with respect to blood flow circulation.

Masaru Ishii (ed.), *Intravital Imaging of Dynamic Bone and Immune Systems: Methods and Protocols*, Methods in Molecular Biology, vol. 1763, https://doi.org/10.1007/978-1-4939-7762-8_13, © Springer Science+Business Media, LLC 2018

We recently established an advanced imaging system to visualize dynamic cell behavior in intravital liver tissues with multiphoton microscopy and quantitatively analyzed their mobility and interactions. Using this system, we assessed the behavior of myeloid cells in the liver of obese mice [2]. We found that the number of rolling and adherent myeloid cells increased significantly, and cell-tracking velocity was decreased in obese mice. We also demonstrated that the blockade of very late antigen-4 (VLA-4), an adhesion molecule, inhibited the transition of myeloid cells from the rolling state to the adhesion state and increased their mean velocity in obese mice. These results suggest that LSECs play an important role in hepatic myeloid cell accumulation via VLA-4-dependent cell-cell adhesion in the fatty liver, resulting in hepatic inflammation and glucose intolerance [2].

In this chapter, we propose the working doses of fluorescent antibodies to stain multiple liver cells in vivo and describe the methodology of intravital multiphoton imaging for visualizing the in vivo behavior of liver cells, as well as their morphology and function in physiological or pathological conditions in the living liver.

2 Materials

2.1 Multiphoton Microscopy

1. Inverted multiphoton microscope (A1R-MP; Nikon).
2. Water-immersion objective, 20× (Plan Fluor: numerical aperture [NA], 0.75; working distance [WD], 0.35 mm; Nikon).
3. Femtosecond-pulsed infrared laser (Chameleon Vision II Ti: sapphire laser; Coherent).
4. External non-descanned detector (NDD) with four channels (Nikon).
5. Dichroic and filter set: three dichroic mirrors (495, 560, and 593 nm) and four band-pass filters (492 nm for the second harmonic generation signal, and Hoechst 33342, 525/50 nm for enhanced green fluorescent protein [EGFP], and fluorescein isothiocyanate [FITC], 575/25 nm for Texas-Red, and 660/52 nm for Qtracker 655; Nikon).
6. NIS Elements integrated software (Nikon).

2.2 Mice and Anesthesia

1. Lysozyme M-EGFP (LysM-EGFP) [3] and wild-type (WT) mice.
2. Isoflurane (Escain).
3. Vaporizer (inhalation device).
4. O_2 bomb.
5. Anesthesia box and mask.

2.3 Intravital Imaging

1. Custom-made stereotactic stage (Fig. 1) (*see* **Note 1**).
2. Shaver and hair removal lotion.
3. Iris scissors and tweezers for mouse surgery.
4. *N*-Butyl cyanoacrylate glue.
5. Infusion line.
6. Infusion syringe pump.
7. Phosphate-buffered saline (PBS), pH 7.4.
8. Electrocardiogram monitoring device.
9. Environmental dark box in which an anesthetized mouse is warmed to 37 °C by an air heater.

2.4 Staining of Blood Vessels, Nuclei, and Cells

1. Angiographic agents: Hoechst 33342, Texas-Red conjugated dextran, Qtracker 655, anti-F4/80-FITC antibody, and anti-CD31-FITC antibody.
2. One 29-gauge insulin syringe for intravenous injection.

2.5 Image Processing and Analysis

1. Image processing and analysis software: Imaris (Bitplane), or NIS Elements (Nikon).
2. After Effects software (Adobe).

3 Methods

3.1 Administration of Fluorescent Dyes

3.1.1 Administration of Fluorescent Antibodies

1. Dissolve anti-F4/80-FITC or anti-CD31-FITC antibody in PBS (*see* **Note 2**).
2. All procedures in mice are performed under anesthesia.
3. Inject anti-F4/80-FITC or anti-CD31-FITC antibody intravenously into mice 2 h before imaging.
4. Perform intravital liver imaging experiments (*see* Subheading 3.2).

3.1.2 Administration of Qtracker 655 and Hoechst 33342

1. Dissolve Qtracker 655 and Hoechst 33342 in PBS (*see* **Note 3**).
2. Inject Qtracker 655 and Hoechst 33342 intravenously into mice immediately before imaging.

3.2 Intravital Multiphoton Imaging of the Liver

1. Initiate the multiphoton microscope and turn on the heater in the environmental dark box.
2. All surgical procedures are performed under isoflurane inhalation anesthesia.
3. Shave the hair and apply hair removal lotion just under the xiphoid process of the mouse.
4. Disinfect the skin of the abdomen using 70% ethanol.
5. Cut the skin and peritoneum minimally using iris scissors and expose the left lobe of the liver (*see* **Note 4**).

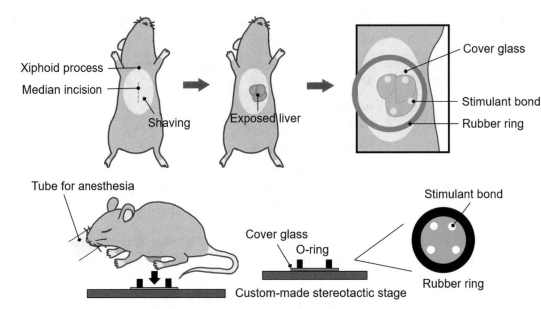

Fig. 1 Schematic illustration of liver imaging. The mouse is anesthetized with isoflurane, the left lobe of the liver is surgically exposed, and the liver is immobilized using the custom-made stereotactic stage

6. Insert a piece of folded gauze between the liver and body of the mouse (*see* **Note 5**).

7. Apply *n*-butyl cyanoacrylate glue to four spots on the cover glass (*see* **Note 6**).

8. Gently place the liver on the cover glass of the custom-made holder (Fig. 1) (*see* **Note 7**).

9. Place the mouse in the environmental dark box.

10. Focus on the liver at an appropriate depth and look through the ocular lenses using a mercury lamp as the light source.

11. Change the light source from the mercury lamp to the Ti: sapphire laser.

12. Set the excitation wavelength, zoom ratio, z-positions, interval time, and duration time using the microscope software (*see* **Note 8**).

13. Observe the internal surface of the liver by multiphoton excitation microscopy (Figs. 2, 3, and 4).

14. Monitor the heart rate of the mouse using an electrocardiogram throughout imaging.

3.3 Image Processing and Analysis

3.3.1 Analysis of Intravital Multiphoton Images

1. Correct images for XY drift using NIS Elements or Imaris software.

2. Analyze images by measuring the frequency and duration of cell-to-cell contacts using Imaris software.

3. Create a movie using After Effects software.

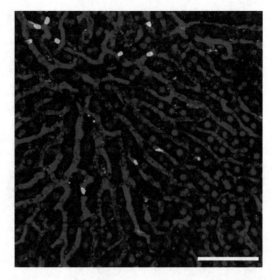

Fig. 2 Visualization of cellular dynamics in the living liver using intravital multi-photon microscopy. Representative images of the liver of LysM-EGFP mice. Green, neutrophils expressing enhanced green fluorescent protein (EGFP); red, blood vessels; blue, nuclei. Scale bar, 100 μm

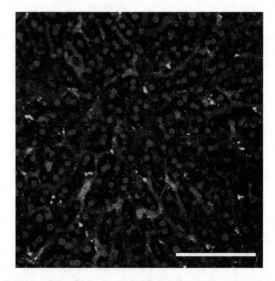

Fig. 3 Visualization of Kupffer cells in the living liver using intravital multiphoton microscopy. Representative images of the liver of wild-type (WT) mice treated with anti-F4/80-fluorescein isothiocyanate (FITC) antibody. Green, Kupffer cells expressing F4/80-FITC; red, blood vessels; blue, nuclei. Scale bar, 100 μm

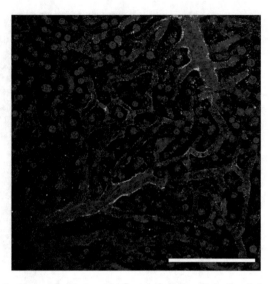

Fig. 4 Visualization of liver sinusoidal endothelial cells in the living liver using intravital multiphoton microscopy. Representative images of the liver of WT mice treated with anti-CD31-FITC antibody. Green, liver sinusoidal endothelial cells expressing CD31-FITC; red, blood vessels; blue, nuclei. Scale bar, 100 μm

4   Notes

1. A commercially available stage with a 24-mm hole is customized on which a cover glass and a 13-mm rubber ring are attached in order from the bottom.
2. To stain Kupffer cells, 100 μl of anti-F4/80-FITC antibody (0.5 mg/ml) can be used and 100 μl of anti-CD31-FITC antibody (0.5 mg/ml) can be used to stain sinusoidal endothelial cells [4].
3. To stain the vascular lumen, 20 μl of Qtracker 655 (or 100 μl of 2 mg/ml Texas-Red conjugated dextran) can be used and 40 μl of 10 mg/ml Hoechst 33342 can be used to stain cell nuclei.
4. The median and left lobes are naturally protruded by pushing bilateral abdomen with hands.
5. A piece of gauze is moistened and inserted between the left lobe and the body of mouse.
6. A small amount of glue is applied to four spots on the glass, forming a trapezoid using the pipette. It is important to prevent drifting of the visual field.
7. The lower edge of the mouse liver should be placed inside the rubber ring as gently as possible.
8. The excitation wavelength of 840 nm is used. For an example of intravital time-lapse liver imaging, image stacks were collected at 5-μm vertical steps at a depth of 40–50 μm below the liver surface, 512 × 512 X–Y resolution, and a time resolution of 1 min.

References

1. Vollmar B, Menger MD (2009) The hepatic microcirculation: mechanistic contributions and therapeutic targets in liver injury and repair. Physiol Rev 89:1269–1339

2. Miyachi Y et al (2017) Roles for cell-cell adhesion and contact in obesity-induced hepatic myeloid cell accumulation and glucose intolerance. Cell Rep 18:2766–2779

3. Faust N et al (2000) Insertion of enhanced green fluorescent protein into the lysozyme gene creates mice with green fluorescent granulocytes and macrophages. Blood 96:719–726

4. Marques PE et al (2015) Imaging liver biology in vivo using conventional confocal microscopy. Nat Protoc 10:258–268

Chapter 14

Intravital Imaging of the Heart at the Cellular Level Using Two-Photon Microscopy

Ryohei Matsuura, Shigeru Miyagawa, Junichi Kikuta, Masaru Ishii, and Yoshiki Sawa

Abstract

Recent molecular approaches have provided deeper insight on heart failure. However, real-time in vivo cellular dynamics have not been satisfactorily visualized. Here, we present a detailed protocol for in vivo cellular imaging for visualization of the rat heart using two-photon microscopy.

Key words Intravital imaging, Two-photon microscopy, Heart, Cardiac tissue, Cardiomyocyte

1 Introduction

Recent advancements in intravital microscopy have clarified dynamic biological events at the cellular level in various healthy and pathological native tissue environments [1–4]. However, real-time (live) in vivo cellular imaging of the beating heart has not been demonstrated to date. Previous studies [5–7] have developed a system for in vivo cellular imaging of the mouse heart using a unique tissue stabilizer and an acquisition-gating method; however, this approach is limited by the requirement for cardiac pacing or retrospective image reconstruction. In addition, the quality of the reported video was insufficient to observe the motion of sarcomere structures in the cardiac myocytes, or blood flow in the surrounding vascular networks. Motion compensation and cardiac tissue stabilization are two of the major practical challenges related to the use of intravital microscopy for imaging physiological and pathological beating hearts.

In this study, we developed a two-photon microscopy system equipped with a custom-built cardiac tissue stabilizer (Fig. 1) facilitated by cardiothoracic surgery for imaging a beating heart in vivo. Using this system, we successfully recorded real-time, clear, hours-long subcellular videos of beating rat hearts. In combination with

Masaru Ishii (ed.), *Intravital Imaging of Dynamic Bone and Immune Systems: Methods and Protocols*, Methods in Molecular Biology, vol. 1763, https://doi.org/10.1007/978-1-4939-7762-8_14, © Springer Science+Business Media, LLC 2018

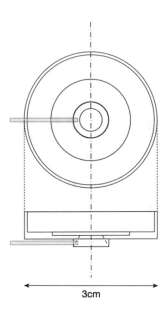

Fig. 1 Stabilizer design. The central hole was cut with an 8-mm diameter and a 1-mm depth and then completely countersunk at a 50° angle to the plane of the stabilizer. The central hole was covered by a round cover glass. A suction tube accessed the chamber through the lateral wall of the central hole, which protruded slightly above the plane of the stabilizer. It attached to the surface of the heart by suction

fluorescent reporter technologies that provide molecular-pathway-specific readouts, this system achieved subcellular spatial resolution and millisecond temporal resolution in beating rat hearts. Thus, we demonstrate intravital imaging of beating cardiac tissue in rats, clearly visualizing contraction and relaxation of the sarcomere structures of individual cardiac myocytes, the distribution of mitochondria in the cardiac myocytes, and blood flow in capillaries under nonischemic conditions. In addition, dynamic changes in each component under pathological conditions such as ischemia can be documented in videos and still images.

2   Materials

2.1   Animals

Adult CAG/GFP transgenic Lewis rats (weighing 250–400 g, male and female) were used, leveraging a previously described transgenic animal technique [8] that ubiquitously expresses the green fluorescence protein (GFP) gene under the control of the CAG promoter.

2.2   Reagents

1. Fluorescence dyes: Alexa Fluor® 568 isolectin GS-IB$_4$ conjugate; Dextran, Texas Red®, 70,000 MW, Neutral; Dextran, Cascade Blue®, 10,000 MW, Anionic, Lysine Fixable; Tetramethylrhodamine, Ethyl Ester, Perchlorate.

2. Phosphate-buffered saline (PBS): 210.0 mg/L KH$_2$PO$_4$, 9000 mg/L NaCl, 726.0 mg/L Na$_2$HPO$_4$·7H$_2$O.

2.3 Equipment

1. Upright multiphoton microscope (A1-MP; Nikon) (*see* **Note 1**).

2. Water-immersion objective, 25× (APO: numerical aperture [NA], 1.0; working distance [WD], 2.0 mm; Nikon).

3. Femtosecond-pulsed infrared laser (Chameleon Vision II Ti:sapphire laser; coherent).

4. External non-descanned detector (NDD) with four channels (Nikon).

5. Fluorescent signals were detected through bandpass emission filters at 492 nm (for blue-labeled dextran), at 525/50 nm (for GFP), and at 629/53 nm (for 70 kDa red-labeled dextran, Alexa Fluor 568-conjugated isolectin B4, and TMRE) (Nikon) (*see* **Note 2**).

6. NIS Elements integrated software (Nikon).

2.4 Intravital Imaging

1. Custom-made stainless-steel plate (Fig. 2) (*see* **Note 3**).

2. Ventilator (Respirator) and ventilation line.

3. Custom-made stabilizer (Fig. 1) (*see* **Note 4**).

4. Iris scissors and tweezers for rat surgery.

5. Infusion line.

6. Phosphate-buffered saline (PBS) buffer, pH 7.4.

7. Electrocardiogram monitoring device.

8. Environmental dark box in which an anesthetized rat is warmed to 37 °C by an air heater.

3 Methods

3.1 Surgical preparation

1. Start the multiphoton microscope and turn on the heater in the environmental dark box (*see* **Note 5**).

2. All procedures in rats should be performed under anesthesia via inhalation of 2% isoflurane, with mechanical ventilation using an endotracheally intubated 18-gauge plastic tube (3-mL tidal volume, 50 times/min).

3. Completely resect the anterior thoracic wall with careful hemostasis using bipolar scissors, then follow with a longitudinal incision of the pericardium to expose the left ventricle (LV) (*see* **Note 6**).

4. Insert a 24-gauge needle into the right jugular vein to allow reagent injection.

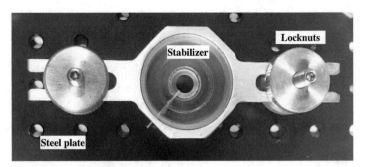

Fig. 2 Experimental setup of the stabilizer and plate. After optimizing the height of the stabilizer from the steel plate, it was fixed in place by tightening locknuts on the bilateral arms via two threaded pillars protruding from the plate

3.2 Intravital Multiphoton Imaging of Cardiac Tissue

1. Inject the fluorescent probe.

2. Place a cover glass attached to a custom-made cardiac stabilizer over the anterior LV wall of the rat.

3. Affix a stabilizer to the custom-made stainless-steel plate using two locknuts, and then immobilize the rat as tightly as possible to avoid drift secondary to respiration and pulsation (*see* **Note 7**) (Fig. 3).

4. Place the rat in the environmental dark box (*see* **Note 8**).

5. Focus on the cardiac tissue at an appropriate depth and look through the ocular lenses using a mercury lamp as the light source.

6. Change the light source from the mercury lamp to the Ti:sapphire laser.

7. Set the excitation wavelength, zoom ratio, z-positions, interval time, and duration time using the microscope software.

8. Observe the cardiac tissue by multiphoton excitation microscopy (Fig. 4).

9. Monitor the heart rate of the rat using an electrocardiogram throughout imaging.

3.3 Image Processing and Analysis

1. Correct image drifts using image-analysis software.

2. The system acquires three-color images (512×512 pixels) at 15 frames/s. The images shall be displayed in real time on a computer monitor and recorded to a hard disk. Raw imaging data are to be processed with the NIS Elements software (Nikon Instruments).

3. Analyze images by measuring the frequency, cell area, and duration of vascular width using NIS Elements.

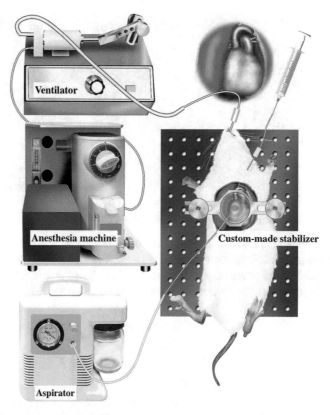

Fig. 3 Schematic illustration of heart imaging. The rat is anesthetized with isoflurane, the front of chest wall is surgically exposed, and its heart is immobilized using the custom-made stabilizer. The equipment included a ventilator, an anesthesia machine, an aspirator, a laser-scanning microscope and a water-dipping objective lens

4   Notes

1. There are two types of microscope: upright and inverted. We believe cardiac tissue can be better observed using an upright microscope. Multiphoton microscopes are also available from other manufacturers (e.g., Leica Microsystems and Olympus).

2. The dichroic and filter set required depend on the fluorescent proteins and dyes used.

3. The custom-made stainless-steel plate is composed of a 10-mm-thick plate, on which two screws with locknuts are placed. The stabilizer can be fixed by tightening its locknuts on its bilateral legs. The height of the stabilizer should be optimized to avoid overly compressing the heart.

4. The stabilizer has one central hole onto which a cover glass is placed. The anterior wall of the heart is affixed gently by suction to the central hole of the stabilizer.

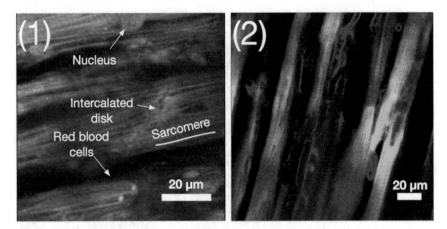

Fig. 4 Real-time in vivo imaging of normal heart beating with the two-photon microscopy system. Regular motion of intercellular connections between adjacent cardiac myocytes (Green, GFP) and blood flow through the capillaries and venules are clearly visualized (1). Blood flow is stained with red-labeled dextran; (2) the endothelium of the microvasculature is stained with red-labeled isolectin B4. Scale bar: 20 μm

5. Some time is required for the laser and temperature to stabilize.

6. Bleeding from internal thoracic arteries should be stopped by an electric knife.

7. The suction pressure should be maintained as low as possible to avoid heart injury due to aspiration. It is also available for mice if the central hole is made smaller.

8. Fix lines to the plate by tape as much as possible to retain connections with the body in the dark box.

References

1. Ishii M, Egen JG, Klauschen F, Meier-Schellersheim M, Saeki Y, Vacher J, Proia RL, Germain RN (2009) Sphingosine-1-phosphate mobilizes osteoclast precursors and regulates bone homeostasis. Nature 458:524–528

2. Kikuta J, Wada Y, Kowada T, Wang Z, Sun-Wada GH, Nishiyama I, Mizukami S, Maiya N, Yasuda H, Kumanogoh A, Kikuchi K, Germain RN, Ishii M (2013) Dynamic visualization of RANKL and Th17-mediated osteoclast function. J Clin Invest 123:866–873

3. Sekimoto R, Fukuda S, Maeda N, Tsushima Y, Matsuda K, Mori T, Nakatsuji H, Nishizawa H, Kishida K, Kikuta J, Maijima Y, Funahashi T, Ishii M, Shimomura I (2015) Visualized macrophage dynamics and significance of S100A8 in obese fat. Proc Natl Acad Sci U S A 112:E2058–E2066

4. Nishikawa K, Iwamoto Y, Kobayashi Y, Katsuoka F, Kawaguchi S, Tsujita T, Nakamura T, Kato S, Yamamoto M, Takayanagi H, Ishii M (2015) DNA methyltransferase 3a regulates osteoclast differentiation by coupling to an S-adenosylmethionine-producing metabolic pathway. Nat Med 21:281–287

5. Lee S, Vinegoni C, Feruglio PF, Fexon L, Gorbatov R, Pivoravov M, Sbarbati A, Nahrendorf M, Weissleder R (2012) Real-time in vivo imaging of the beating mouse heart at microscopic resolution. Nat Commun 3:1054

6. Aguirre AD, Vinegoni C, Sebas M, Weissleder R (2014) Intravital imaging of cardiac function at the single-cell level. Proc Natl Acad Sci U S A 111:11257–11262

7. Vinegoni C, Aguirre AD, Lee S, Weissleder R (2015) Imaging the beating heart in the mouse using intravital microscopy techniques. Nat Protoc 10:1802–1819

8. Inoue H, Ohsawa I, Murakami T, Kimura A, Hakamata Y, Sato Y, Kaneko T, Takahashi M, Okada T, Ozawa K, Francis J, Leone P, Kobayashi E (2005) Development of new inbred transgenic strains of rats with LacZ or GFP. Biochem Biophys Res Commun 329:288–295

Chapter 15

Imaging Window Device for Subcutaneous Implantation Tumor

Wataru Ikeda, Ken Sasai, and Tsuyoshi Akagi

Abstract

Most of preclinical cancer studies use xenograft models established from human cell lines or patient-derived cancer cells subcutaneously implanted into the flank of immunocompromised mice. These models are often assumed to represent the original diseases and are valuable tools, at least to some extent, for understanding both the basic biology of cancer and for proof-of-concept studies of molecularly targeted therapies. However, analyzing the cellular behavior of individual components within xenografts, including tumor cells, stromal cells, immune cells, and blood vessels, is challenging. In particular, it has been difficult and urgently required to trace the whole process of heterogeneous tumor microenvironment formation mediated by various components described above. Here we demonstrate a method for monitoring this process using a window device system that we have recently developed and a subcutaneous xenograft model that accurately recapitulates the histology of human lung adenocarcinoma. Use of our imaging window device and a multiphoton laser scanning microscope provides a powerful tool for investigating tumor heterogeneity and responses to drug treatments in an in vivo live imaging system.

Key words Subcutaneous implantation tumor, Repeatability of microscopic field, Intravital imaging, Multiphoton laser scanning microscope, Angiogenesis, Anticancer reagent, Cancer immunology

1 Introduction

Intravital microscopy performed on window device preparations or through the skin on tissues enables non/low-invasive, high resolution studies of tumor pathophysiology [1–3]. Although transillumination and fluorescence microscopy are widely employed techniques, these techniques do not provide 3D information and have a relatively low penetration depth. By contrast, confocal and multiphoton laser scanning microscopy enable high-resolution 3D imaging and multiparametric recording. Using high numerical aperture objectives, lateral resolutions of approximately 250 nm can be obtained. Various window devices have been developed for intravital microscopy imaging of developing tumors; these devices include a cranial imaging window [4], dorsal skinfold chamber [5, 6], mammary imaging window [7, 8], and abdominal imaging

Masaru Ishii (ed.), *Intravital Imaging of Dynamic Bone and Immune Systems: Methods and Protocols*, Methods in Molecular Biology, vol. 1763, https://doi.org/10.1007/978-1-4939-7762-8_15, © Springer Science+Business Media, LLC 2018

window [9, 10]. Although these window devices have proven extremely valuable, further improvement is required. These window systems can be used in studies lasting days to months; however, ensuring the repeatability of a microscopic field on an arbitrary day is a technical challenge. Therefore, many researchers applied various strategies to ensure the imaging of the same microscopic field [3]. Many imaging windows are made of solid metal to maintain the shape for a long time; however using metal also makes the window heavy and causes the mouse a lot of stress. In particular, the shape of the dorsal skinfold chamber [5, 6] could hinder the natural behavior of a mouse. To resolve these issues, we used polymethylmethacrylate (PMMA) to produce the window frame, which makes the device lighter than those made of solid metal. Furthermore, our window frame enables a tight connection to the hole of the stage insert in a multiphoton laser scanning microscope system and enables the consistent reproducibility of the microscopic field throughout an experiment with the same mouse using guides marked on the window frame and microscope stage. Here, we provide a method for monitoring the progression of a tumor [subcutaneous implantation lung adenocarcinoma model (HSAEC-4T53RD cells); *see* ref. 11 for detail] using our new window device and multiphoton laser scanning microscopy. Because the xenografts derived from the HSAEC-4T53RD cells comprise malignant glandular epithelial cells and fibrous stroma [11], time-dependent changes in tumor growth and tumor vessel structures can be comprehensively demonstrated (*see* Fig. 5). With the availability of high-resolution microscopes, molecular probes, and suitable xenograft models, the imaging system described here would be applicable for monitoring tumor heterogeneity, angiogenesis, and therapeutic responses at a molecular level.

2   Materials

2.1   Subcutaneous Imaging Window (SIW)

1. Custom-made SIW made of polymethylmethacrylate (PMMA) (*see* Fig. 1a, b, *see* **Note 1**).
2. 10-mm circular glass coverslip.
3. Cyanoacrylate glue.
4. Milli-Q ultrapurified water.
5. 70% ethanol.

2.2   Subcutaneous Implantation of Imaging Window Device

1. 4–6-week-old female immune deficient mice (e.g., nude, SCID, etc.).
2. Animal shaver.
3. Depilatory cream.
4. Cotton swab (sterilized, if possible).

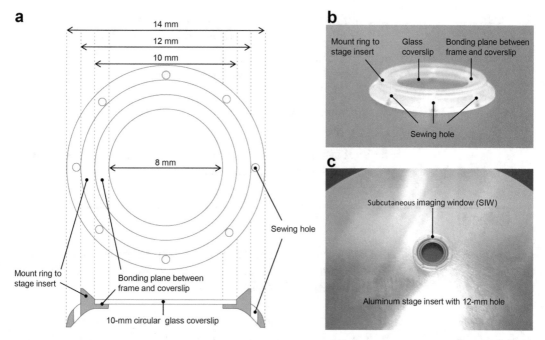

Fig. 1 Subcutaneous imaging window (SIW). (**a**) Schematic top view (upper) and simplified cross-sectional view (bottom) of the SIW. (**b**) Components of the SIW and the name of each part. (**c**) The SIW placed into the hole of the stage insert of the microscope

5. Kim towel (sterilized, if possible).

6. Cultured tumor cells (e.g., HSAEC 4T53RD cells, *see* ref. 11, *see* **Note 2**).

7. Culture medium (appropriate for cultured tumor cells, e.g., SAGM Bullet Kit (Lonza) for HSAEC 4T53RD cells)

8. Trypsin.

9. PBS(−).

10. Corning® Matrigel®, growth factor reduced, phenol-red free.

11. Isoflurane and anesthetics machine.

12. Devon™ Surgical skin marker.

13. Round ruler (10-mm).

14. Spring scissors, straight, 10 cm.

15. Extra fine graefe forceps, 10 cm.

16. Micro needle holder.

17. Nonabsorbable thread with needle.

2.3 Maintenance of the Mice

1. Sterile cotton gauze.

2. 3 M™ Tegaderm™ Transparent Film Roll.

3. Baby lotion.

2.4 Imaging	1. Multiphoton laser scanning microscope system A1R MP+ with GaAsP NDD and inverted microscope TiE (A1R MP+, NIKON).

2. Custom-made aluminum stage insert with 12-mm hole (*see* Fig. 1c, *see* **Note 3**).

3. Specimen clips.

4. Micro serrefines.

5. Vital sign monitor with body temperature controller (e.g., PhysioSuite®, Kent Scientific).

3   Methods

All animal studies were performed with the approval of the Animal Ethics Committee at KAN Research Institute according to Laboratory Animal Welfare guidelines.

3.1   Preparation of Subcutaneous Imaging Window (SIW)

1. Wash the SIW frame with 70% ethanol and allow to dry.

2. Adhere a 10-mm circular glass coverslip to the SIW using cyanoacrylate glue (*see* Fig. 1b, *see* **Note 4**).

3. Wait for 15 min (*see* **Note 5**).

4. Wash the SIW with Milli-Q ultrapurified water.

5. Wash the SIW with 70% ethanol (*see* **Note 6**).

6. Sterilize the SIW by UV exposure for 3 h on each side on a clean bench.

7. Store the SIW in a sterilized cell culture dish.

3.2   Preimplantation Preparation of Imaging Window Device with Cultured Tumor Cells

The following operations (**steps 1** and **5** in Subheadings 3.2) are performed on a clean bench or a biological safety cabinet.

1. Trypsinize the cultured tumor cells, wash the cells with PBS($-$), and prepare the tumor cell suspension in 50% Matrigel® in culture medium (e.g., 1×10^7 cells/ml) (*see* **Note 7**).

2. Place a drop (e.g., 10 μl) of the tumor cell suspension on the coverslip of the SIW (*see* Fig. 2, *see* **Note 8**).

3. Incubate the SIW for 5 min at 37 °C in a CO_2 incubator.

4. Coat the drop of tumor cell suspension with Matrigel® (e.g., 150 μl).

5. Incubate the SIW for 15 min at 37 °C in a CO_2 incubator.

6. Place the SIW on a heat block at 30–37 °C until implantation.

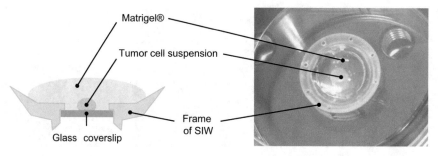

Fig. 2 Preparation of the SIW with cultured tumor cells. Approximately 10 μl (one drop) of tumor cell suspension in 50% Matrigel® should first be placed on the coverslip of the device, and then Matrigel® should be overlaid. See the Methods for details

3.3 Subcutaneous
Implantation
of the SIW

The following operations are performed in a SPF clean room (or on a clean bench).

1. Anesthetize a mouse in an induction chamber using 2.5% (vol/vol) isoflurane.

2. Place the anesthetized mouse on a Kim towel and continue the administration of anesthesia using 1.5% (vol/vol) isoflurane via a nose cone.

3. Remove hair between the foreleg and the hind leg of the mouse using a small animal shaver.

4. Remove the rest of the hair using depilatory cream (*see* **Note 9**).

5. Wash the skin with warm tap water and dry the body using a Kim towel.

6. Place the unconscious mouse on a Kim towel and continue the administration of anesthesia using 1.5% (vol/vol) isoflurane via a nose cone (*see* **Note 10**).

7. Sterilize the skin with 70% ethanol.

8. Draw a straight line along the backbone and then draw a 10-mm circle 5 mm away from the straight line using a skin marker (*see* Fig. 3a, *see* **Note 11**).

9. Cut out the skin along the outside of the circle using spring scissors and extra fine graefe forceps (*see* Fig. 3b).

10. Place the SIW containing the tumor cells (prepared in Subheading 3.3) in the area where the skin has been removed (*see* Fig. 3c).

11. Pull the edge of skin around the SIW and put it on top of the outer ring (*see* Fig. 3d).

12. Suture the skin to the SIW using the holes in the SIW and nonabsorbable thread with a needle and micro needle holder, and tie using a surgical knot (*see* Fig. 3e, *see* **Note 12**).

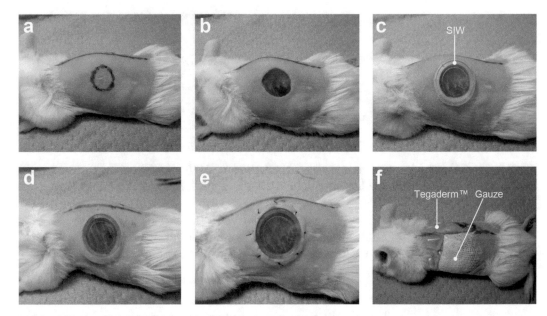

Fig. 3 Surgical procedure. (**a**) The straight line along the backbone and the 10-mm circle. The circle is located 5-mm away from the backbone line. (**b**) A hole for placing the SIW, after removal of the 10-mm circle of mouse skin. (**c**) The SIW placed on the skin hole. The SIW has an appropriate number of tumor cells in Matrigel® (*see* Fig. 2). (**d**, **e**) Procedures for anchoring the device. See the Methods for details. (**f**) After surgery, mice should be maintained with cotton gauze and Tegaderm™ Transparent Film Roll, as indicated, to protect the device from damage and/or breakdown

3.4 Maintenance of the Mice

1. Place sterile cotton gauze (approximately 1-cm square) on the SIW and wrap the body and the SIW in Tegaderm™ Transparent Film Roll (cut into 3.5-cm wide strips) (*see* Fig. 3f, *see* **Note 13**).

2. Keep the mouse individually in a cage (*see* **Note 14**).

3. Exchange the gauze and Tegaderm™ twice a week for the period of keeping the mouse (*see* **Notes 15–17**).

4. If necessary, record into the status of the SIW using the digital device, such as a compact digital camera, a stereo microscope equipped with a CCD camera, etc. (*see* **Note 18**).

3.5 Image Acquisition

1. Anesthetize the mouse in an induction chamber using 2.5% (vol/vol) isoflurane.

2. Place the unconscious mouse on a Kim towel and continue the administration of anesthesia using 1.5% (vol/vol) isoflurane via a nose cone.

3. Remove the gauze and Tegaderm™ from the mouse.

4. Thoroughly clean the glass using 70% ethanol and a cotton swab until it is completely transparent.

5. For visualizing something (e.g., blood, nuclei, etc.), appropriate imaging agent(s) are injected intravenously via the tail vein or retro orbital sinus (*see* **Note 19**).

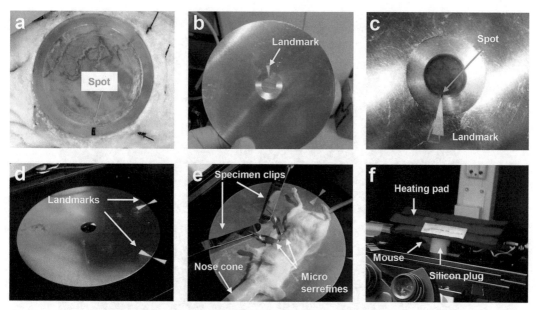

Fig. 4 Setup for intravital imaging. (**a–c**) Guides should be marked on the mount ring of the SIW (**a**, spot) and on the edge of stage insert hole (**b**, landmark) for continuous investigation. These guides function as landmarks for observation area by adjusting them as indicated in **c**. (**d**) The stage insert should be placed on the microscope stage by aligning the position using landmarks marked on the stage and on the outer ring of the stage insert. (**e**) Typical appearance of a mouse placed on the stage of the microscope. Specimen clips and micro serrefines should be used as indicated. (**f**) A mouse under microscope imaging. A heating pad should be used for maintaining the body temperature

6. For the first observation, mark the spot (landmark) on the mount ring of the SIW using a permanent marker (*see* Fig. 4a, *see* **Note 20**).

7. Mount the SIW onto the aluminum stage insert and align to the appropriate position using the landmark (*see* Fig. 4b, c).

8. Place the stage insert onto the stage of the microscope and align to the correct position using the landmarks on the stage insert and the stage (*see* Fig. 4d, e, *see* **Note 21**).

9. Anesthetize the mouse on the stage using 0.5–1.5% (vol/vol) isoflurane via a nose cone (*see* Fig. 4e, *see* **Note 22**).

10. Hold the SIW and surrounding skin using specimen clips extended with micro serrefines (*see* Fig. 4e, *see* **Note 23**).

11. Measure vital signs and regulate the body temperature of the mouse using PhysioSuite® (*see* Fig. 4f, *see* **Note 24**).

12. Acquire fluorescence images [such as 2D (x–y), 3D (x–y–z), timelapse (x–y–t), and 4D (x–y–z–t)] using a multiphoton laser scanning microscope (*see* Fig. 5a, b, *see* **Note 25** and **26**).

13. After observation, maintain the mouse according to Subheading 3.4 (*see* **Note 27**).

14. Repeat imaging on the scheduled day (*see* Fig. 5b, *see* **Note 28**).

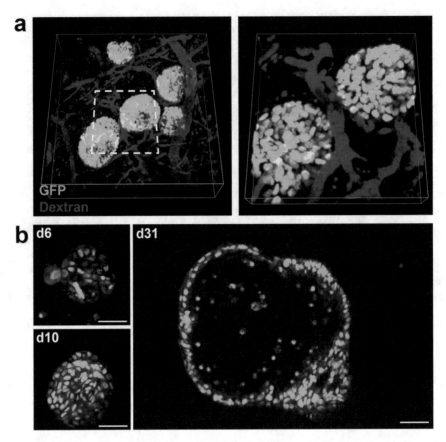

Fig. 5 Observation of xenograft tumor growing under the SIW using a multiphoton laser scanning microscope. (**a**) Typical image of subcutaneous xenograft tumor under the window device. GFP (green) indicates nuclei of HSAEC-4T53RD cells. Distance between tumor cells (green nuclei) and tumor vessels (red, TRITC-conjugated dextran) can be monitored. Labeled dextran was intravenously injected prior to imaging. High magnification image (right panel) enables the investigation of the interaction between tumor cells and vessels. *x*, *y*, and *z* are 516, 516, and 136 µm, respectively, in the left panel. *x*, *y*, and *z* are 201, 201, and 38 µm, respectively, in the right panel. (**b**) Time-dependent tumor growth under the SIW. Identical tumor cells were continuously analyzed by taking images at the same position under the SIW (6, 10, and 31 days after implantation, as indicated). Tumor development can be monitored by observing the increased area around the cell with green nuclei. Cavity within the ring of green cells represents the lumen of a glandular structure. Scale bars, 50 µm

4   Notes

1. STEM Biomethod Co. (Fukuoka, Japan, http://stem-biomethod.co.jp/) provided the custom-made SIW upon our request. This device has a mount ring to the stage plate. The mount ring enables a tight-connection with 12-mm hole on the aluminum stage insert (*see* Subheading 2.4, **item 2** and *see* Fig. 1c).

2. When a fluorescence protein or its fusion protein is exogenously expressed in the tumor cells, its labeling is very useful for identification and tracing etc. We usually use a nuclear-

localized fluorescence protein, such as GFP fused to H2B, to identify a single cell.

3. STEM Biomethod Co. (Fukuoka, Japan, http://stem-biomethod.co.jp/) provided the custom-made aluminum stage insert with a 12-mm hole upon our request.

4. Place the circular glass coverslip on the bonding plane of the SIW, and then pour the glue into the interspace between the coverslip and the SIW. Using a needle nozzle for the glue would be convenient.

5. Wipe the window with acetone using a cotton swab in case misty spots appear owing to vapor from the glue.

6. Use a cotton swab to clean the glass so that it is completely transparent.

7. Matrigel® and its mixture are handled while cooling it on ice to avoid stiffening.

8. The SIW is placed into a sterile culture dish for transport.

9. Depilation treatment may be performed one day before transplantation. Depilation treatment is not necessary for nude mice.

10. Warm the mouse using a heating pad to maintain its body temperature during surgery.

11. Usually, we implant the SIW on left flank (on the spleen side).

12. Eight sutures are necessary to secure the SIW to the skin flap. Regarding the order of needlework, one place is sutured and then the opposite place is sutured.

13. This procedure is very useful to secure the SIW and to retain the skin's moisture.

14. Keeping two or more mice in a cage causes damage to the SIW. If necessary, provide an antibiotic mixture (such as sulfamethoxazole and trimethoprim) and/or anti-inflammatory drugs (such as carprofen or dexamethasone) for 3 days after the surgery.

15. If the skin is dirty, clean it with a wet cotton swab or surgical cotton. If the surgical skin edge is dry, put a small amount of baby lotion on it.

16. If the hair grows back at the depilated area, shave again using a small animal shaver. Do not use depilatory cream.

17. If the SIW and mouse are carefully kept, this system can be maintained for up to 2 months.

18. Most tumor cells undergo angiogenesis during tumor formation. Therefore, in many cases, bleeding is observed 3–7 days after implantation. The bleeding causes interference during

fluorescence microscopy observation, but the bleeding is usually absorbed 1–2 weeks after implantation.

19. We usually use fluorophore-conjugated dextran (MW 100–200 kDa) to visualize blood, and Hoechst 33342 to visualize nuclei of blood cells and tissues.

20. This spot is very important for repeatability of the microscopic field.

21. The repeatability of the microscopic field depends on Subheading 3.5 **steps 6** and **7** and on using a motorized stage with a coordinate recognition function.

22. Subheading 3.5 **steps 7–9** should be promptly executed while the anesthetic is at its most effective.

23. Although an inverted microscope is useful for reducing tissue movement caused by respiration, this treatment is effective at preventing imaging distortions.

24. We can check the condition of the anesthetized mouse by monitoring the SpO2 level and heart rate. Regulation of the body temperature prevents hypothermia caused by anesthetizing. The heating pad is supported by silicon plugs to make a gap between the heating pad and the mouse.

25. When acquiring an image, record the coordinate data of the motorized stage. This information is necessary for the repeatability of the microscopic field.

26. If the observation is prolonged, the administration of an appropriate volume (e.g., 0.5 ml) of saline solution in the subcutaneous space of the mouse every 3 h can prevent dehydration.

27. If the imaging system is placed in the SPF clean area as the breeding room, it is possible to perform observations repeatedly on the scheduled day.

28. To obtain the same tumor image, repeat the physical setting, such as alignment of the landmarks, and load the coordinate data of the previous image. If possible, find some inherent landmarks in the microscopic field, such as blood vessels and their pattern, and collagen patterns using second harmonic generation signals. The microscopic field is reproduced with a high probability when following these steps.

References

1. Beerling E, Ritsma L, Vrisekoop N, Derksen PW, van Rheenen J (2011) Intravital microscopy: new insights into metastasis of tumors. J Cell Sci 124:299–310

2. Condeelis J, Weissleder R (2010) In vivo imaging in cancer. Cold Spring Harb Perspect Biol 2:a003848

3. Alieva M, Ritsma L, Giedt RJ, Weissleder R, van Rheenen J (2014) Imaging windows for long-term intravital imaging: general overview and technical insights. Intravital 3:e29917

4. Kienast Y, von Baumgarten L, Fuhrmann M, Klinkert WE, Goldbrunner R, Herms J, Winkler F (2010) Real-time imaging reveals the single steps of brain metastasis formation. Nat Med 16:116–122

5. Gaustad JV, Simonsen TG, Leinaas MN, Rofstad EK (2012) A novel application of dorsal window chambers: repetitive imaging of tumor-associated lymphatics. Microvasc Res 83:360–365

6. Alexander S, Koehl GE, Hirschberg M, Geissler EK, Friedl P (2008) Dynamic imaging of cancer growth and invasion: a modified skin-fold chamber model. Histochem Cell Biol 130:1147–1154

7. Kedrin D, Gligorijevic B, Wyckoff J, Verkhusha VV, Condeelis J, Segall JE, van Rheenen J (2008) Intravital imaging of metastatic behavior through a mammary imaging window. Nat Methods 5:1019–1021

8. Schafer R, Leung HM, Gmitro AF (2014) Multi-modality imaging of a murine mammary window chamber for breast cancer research. BioTechniques 57:45–50

9. Ritsma L, Steller EJ, Beerling E, Loomans CJ, Zomer A, Gerlach C, Vrisekoop N, Seinstra D, van Gurp L, Schafer R, Raats DA, de Graaff A, Schumacher TN, de Koning EJ, Rinkes IH, Kranenburg O, van Rheenen J (2012) Intravital microscopy through an abdominal imaging window reveals a pre-micrometastasis stage during liver metastasis. Sci Transl Med 4:158ra145

10. Ritsma L, Steller EJ, Ellenbroek SI, Kranenburg O, Borel Rinkes IH, van Rheenen J (2013) Surgical implantation of an abdominal imaging window for intravital microscopy. Nat Protoc 8:583–594

11. Sasai K, Sukezane T, Yanagita E, Nakagawa H, Hotta A, Itoh T, Akagi T (2011) Oncogene-mediated human lung epithelial cell transformation produces adenocarcinoma phenotypes in vivo. Cancer Res 71:2541–2549

New Tools for Imaging of Immune Systems: Visualization of Cell Cycle, Cell Death, and Cell Movement by Using the Mice Lines Expressing Fucci, SCAT3.1, and Kaede and KikGR

Michio Tomura

Abstract

Visualization of biological events in real time in vivo has become a crucial to understand immune responses. We have been established novel visualization tools for life of immune cells: proliferation, cell death, and migration. Fucci-transgenic mice allow us to visualize cell cycle phases by reciprocal expression of mKusabira-Orange2 in G_1 phase and mAzami-Green in $S/G_2/M$ phase. Caspase-3 indicator SCAT3.1 knock-in mice visualize cell death by changing color. Photoconvertible proteins, Kaede and KikGR expressing mice track cell movement between organs by labeling immune cells as red color. Here, I will introduce how to use and visualize these mice. These techniques will help to understand immune system in the living whole body.

Key words Cell cycle, Fucci, Photoconvertible protein, Cell migration, Kaede, KikGR, Cell death, Caspase-3, SCAT3.1

1 Introduction

Recently, visualization of biological events in vivo directly using living mice is crucial technique to elucidate immune responses [1, 2]. In addition, clarification of immune cell movement between organs with their phenotype and functions is important to understand the biological roles of immune cells in immune homeostasis. We have been established novel visualization tools for life of immune cells: Fucci-transgenic (Tg) mice for cell cycle phases [3], caspase-3 indicator SCAT3.1 knock-in (KI) mice for cell death [4], and photoconvertible protein, Kaede and KikGR expressing mice for cell movement [5, 6]. In this chapter, I will introduce how to use and visualize these mice with two-photon microcopy, and detect by flow cytometry. However, general information of

Masaru Ishii (ed.), *Intravital Imaging of Dynamic Bone and Immune Systems: Methods and Protocols*, Methods in Molecular Biology, vol. 1763, https://doi.org/10.1007/978-1-4939-7762-8_16, © Springer Science+Business Media, LLC 2018

intravital two-photon laser imaging is not described in this chapter, please follow previously published papers [1, 2].

1.1 Fucci-Tg Mice

Fucci (*f*luorescent *u*biquitination-based *c*ell *c*ycle *i*ndicator) transgenic mice allow us to visualize cell cycle progression in vivo. Fucci utilizes the ubiquitin oscillation of cell cycle transitions control [7]. Fusion proteins monomeric Kusabira-Orange2 (mKO2) with human Cdt1(30/120) (mKO2-hCdt1) and monomeric Azami-Green (mAG) with human Geminin (1/110) (mAG-hGem) accumulate in the nuclei of cells in $G_1(G_0)$ phase (mKO2-positive) and $S/G_2/M$ phase (mAG-positive), reciprocally (Fig. 1a). Thus, G_1 phase in cell cycle cycling cells (lower or negative mKO2 signal) and quiescent G_0 phase (the highest signals of mKO2) can be distinguished (Fig. 1b). There are two combinations of transgenic mouse lines using the CAG promoter to drive gene expression of mKO2-hCdt1 or mAG-hGem. A cross-bred mouse line #594/#504 is used for imaging of the cell cycle of neural progenitor cells and other mesenchymal cells [7]. On the other hand, for imaging of hematopoietic lineage cells, a cross-bred mouse line mAG-hGem expressing FucciS/G_2/M-#474 with mKO2-expressing FucciG$_1$-#639 is used, because #596/#504 does not express neither mKO2-hCdt1 nor mAG-hGem in the hematopoietic lineage cells [3].

1.2 SCAT3.1 Mice

Cell death is one of the important events in the immune system. Apoptotic cell death is induced during thymic T cell selection, killing of target infected cells and tumor cells by killer cells. Caspase-3, important enzyme to mediate apoptosis, is activated by both extrinsic pathway such as FAS and intrinsic pathways of apoptosis [8]. Caspase-3 indicator SCAT3.1 is a fusion protein of enhanced cyan fluorescent protein (ECFP), caspase-3 cleavable peptide, and enhanced yellow fluorescent protein (EYFP) analogue Venus. Cleavage of caspase-3 cleavable peptide by active caspase-3 generated by apoptotic signal impairs intramolecular fluorescence resonance energy transfer (FRET) between the two fluorescent proteins

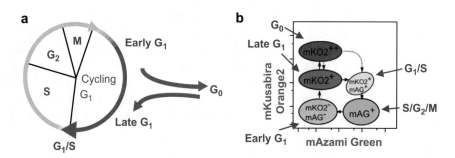

Fig. 1 Visualization of cell cycle phases by Fucci system. (**a**) Exposure of Fucci signals during cell cycle. (**b**) Flow cytometric dot pot of individual cell cycle phases

and changes the emission wavelength (Fig. 2a) [4, 9, 10]. SCAT3.1 mice were generated by cross-mating ROSA26-loxP-stop-loxP-SCAT3.1 mice with CAG-Cre mice in order to delete the loxP-stop-loxP site. Cell type-specific SCAT3.1-expressing mice are achieved by cross-mating ROSA26-loxP-stop-loxP-SCAT3.1 knock-in mice with an appropriate Cre-expressing mouse strains.

Here, I introduce how to use and visualize SCAT3.1 transfected cells in vivo using CTL and target interaction (Fig. 2b).

1.3 Kaede and KikGR Expressing Mice

Photoconvertible proteins Kaede and KikGR are purified from stony corals, and humanized. Fluorescence color of Kaede and KikGR changes irreversibly from green to red upon exposure to violet light (Fig. 3a) [11, 12]. I note that KikGR has considerably

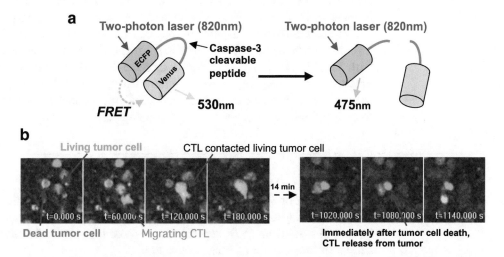

Fig. 2 Visualization of cell death by caspase-3 indicator SCAT3.1. (**a**) Schematic representation of SCAT3.1. (**b**) Detection of CTL tumor killing in vivo. SCAT3.1-expressing tumor cell line was inoculated to Rag2$^{-/-}$ mice, and transferred Cell Tracker Green-labeled CTL. Tumor mass was observed with intravital two-photon microscopy

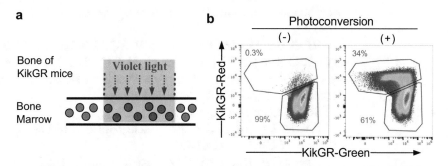

Fig. 3 Photoconversion of bone marrow cells. (**a**) Exposure to violet light changes KikGR color from green to red. (**b**) Flow cytometric dot plots of CD45$^+$ cells from non-photoconverted (−) and immediately after photoconversion (+) with exposure to violet light (436 nm) at 500 mW/cm^2 for 5 min. Percentage in plot indicates percentage of parent population

greater photoconversion efficiency than Kaede [6]. By using Kaede or KikGR expressing mice, after labeling of cells by photoconversion with violet light, we can monitor replacement of cells in photoconverted site and track migratory cells to other anatomical site in the living mice [5, 6]. We and our colleagues have utilized these mice lines and revealed important immunological roles with their movement [5, 6, 13–18]. Photoconversion of Kaede and KikGR with two-photon laser and tracking photoconverted cells by intravital microscopy are possible [15].

All of the cells including immune cells express Kaede and KikGR in Kaede-transgenic mice and KikGR mice, respectively. KikGR mice were generated by cross-mating ROSA26-loxP-stop-loxP-KikGR mice with CAG-Cre mice in order to delete the loxP-stop-loxP site [6]. Cell type-specific KikGR-expressing mice are achieved by cross-mating ROSA26-loxP-stop-loxP-KikGR knock-in mice with an appropriate Cre-expressing mouse strains [16].

Here, I introduce a new in vivo cell tracking system for the direct assessment of cell movement from the bone marrow (BM) with KikGR mice [17]. I recommend to see the protocols reported previously for detecting cell replacement within skin and cell movement from skin to other anatomical sites, and of cell movement from inguinal lymph node to the skin using Kaede-Tg mice [19].

2 Materials

2.1 Mice

All mouse strains were deposited in RIKEN BRC. Please contact RIKEN BRC (animal@brc.riken.jp) to obtain these mice with following information. PCR conditions for screening mouse lines are shown in home page of each mouse line.

FucciS/G$_2$/M-#474;   B6.Cg-Tg(FucciS/G2/M)#474Bsi (RBRC02704)   http://www2.brc.riken.jp/lab/animal/detail.php?brc_no=RBRC02704&lang=en (*see* **Note 1**).

FucciG$_1$-#639; B6.Cg-Tg(FucciG1)#639Bsi http://www2.brc.riken.jp/lab/animal/detail.php?reg_no=RBRC02709   (*see* **Note 1**).

ROSA-CAG-loxP-stop-loxP-SCAT3.1mice;B6.B6129-Gt(ROSA)26Sor<tml(CAG-ECFP/Venus) Kgwa>(RBRC04848)   http://www2.brc.riken.jp/lab/animal/detail.php?brc_no=RBRC04848&lang=en.

SCAT3.1 mice; deposit process is ongoing.

Kaede-Tg mice for B6 background; B6.Cg-Tg (CAG-tdKaede)15Utr (RBRC05737).

Kaede-Tg mice for B/c background; C.Cg-Tg (CAG-tdKaede)15Utr (RBRC09257).

ROSA-CAG-loxP-stop-loxP-KikGR   mice; B6.Cg-Gt(ROSA)26Sor<tml(CAG-.kikGR)

Kgwa>(RBRC09254)   http://www2.brc.riken.jp/lab/animal/detail.php?brc_no=RBRC09254&lang=en.

KikGR mice; B6.Cg-Gt(ROSA)26Sor<tm1.1(CAG-kikGR) Kgwa>(RBRC09256)   http://www2.brc.riken.jp/lab/animal/detail.php?brc_no=RBRC09256&lang=en (*see* **Notes 2** and **3**).

2.2 Observation of Cell Cycle Phases and Cell Death by Two-Photon Laser Microscopy

1. Two-photon laser microscopy composed of two-photon laser and following detection filter sets.

2. Detection filter set for Fucci and second harmonic signals (SHG); 495, and 560 nm dichroic mirrors in combination with 492SP (SHG), 525/50 (mAG), and 575/25 (mKO2) nm band-pass filters.

3. Detection filter set for SCAT3.1 and SHG signals; 440 and 510 nm dichroic mirrors in combination with 435SP (SHG), 480/30 (ECFP), and 535/26 (EYFP, and Cell Tracker Green) nm band-pass filters.

4. Cell Tracker Green.

2.3 Flow Cytometry

1. For detection of mAG2, mKO2, non-photoconverted and photoconverted Kaede and KikGR, flow cytometer that is minimum spec to detect FITC and PE (*see* **Notes 4** and **5**).

2. For detection of SCAT3.1, flow cytometer has laser at 405 nm or 440 nm and 510/23 nm and 535/26 nm band-pass filters.

2.4 Photoconversion of Kaede or KikGR

1. Light source: Spot UV curing equipment, SP9 250VB or SP500VB with 436-nm band-pass filter (*see* **Note 6**). Glass fiber unit: (SF-101NQ). Collator: B lens unit (Ushio).

2. UV intensity meter: Digital UV intensity meter UIT-201, Detector: UVD405PD (Ushio).

3. Anesthesia: Isoflurane inhalator

4. Aluminum foil.

5. Antibodies: Appropriate fluorochrome-conjugated (except for FITC, phycoerythrin (PE), and Texas-Red (Tx-Red) or PE-Dazzle954 antibodies for staining cells) (*see* **Note 7**).

3 Methods

3.1 Observation of Cell Cycle Phases by Two-Photon Microscopy

1. Signals of mKO2, mAG, and second harmonic signals (SHG) were excited by two-photon laser light at 930 nm, and emission signals were detected (*see* **Note 8**).

3.2 Observation of Cell Death by Two-Photon Microscopy

1. Signals of SCAT3.1, Cell Tracker Green, and SHG were excited by two-photon laser light at 820 nm, and emission signals were detected (Fig. 2b) (*see* **Note 9**).

3.3 Photoconversion of Bone Marrow Cells in Femur in KikGR Mice

1. Position the detector of UV intensity meter at the exposure point.

2. Adjust the intensity of violet light at the exposure point to 500 mW/cm² by moving up and down the position of the collator or shutter inside the light source.

3. Anesthetize KikGR mouse with isoflurane [ca. 2% (vol/vol)] by inhalation.

4. Cut the skin vertically at the dorsal side of the thigh, and opposite side of thigh (*see* **Notes 10** and **11**).

5. Visualize femur by separating the vastus lateralis and biceps femoris muscles gently (*see* **Note 10**).

6. Hold the muscle to visualize the femur by bone reduction forceps (*see* **Note 12**).

7. Cover the surrounding tissue with aluminum foil.

8. Expose the femur to violet light (436 nm) at 500 mW/cm² for 5 min through a hole in the foil with continuous instillation of warmed PBS (*see* **Note 13**).

9. Replace the muscle surrounding the femur.

10. Close the wound with suture.

3.4 Flow Cytometry Detection of Cell Cycle with Fucci-Tg Mice

1. Prepare BM cells or thymocytes, and lymphocytes from lymph node or spleen (*see* **Note 14**).

2. These cells are subjected to flow cytometer.

3. Set voltages to detect mKO2 signal and mAG signal.

4. Acquire data of samples.

3.5 Flow Cytometry Detection of Cell Death with SCAT3.1 Mice

1. Prepare living cells and dead cells of SCAT3.1-expressing cells (*see* **Note 15**).

2. Living cells and dead cells of SCAT3.1-expressing cells are subjected to flow cytometer.

3. Set voltages to detect ECFP signal and Venus signal.

4. Acquire data of samples (*see* **Note 16**).

3.6 Flow Cytometry Detection of Cell Movement with Kaede or KikGR Mice

1. Prepare non-photoconverted and photoconverted cells those were stained with appropriate mAbs (*see* **Note 17**).

2. Adjust the intensities of Kaede and KikGR signals in FITC and PE channels to three-fourths of the total range using the lymphocytes from Kaede and KikGR mice.

3. Acquire data of samples.

4. Immediately after photoconversion as described in Subheading 3.3, 34% of CD45+ gated BM cells were photoconverted (Fig. 3b and *see* **Notes 17** and **18**).

4   Notes

1. You can visualize both $S/G_2/M$ and G_1 phase in one cell after cross-mating FucciS/G_2/M-#474 mice and FucciG$_1$-#639 mice. Visualization of $S/G_2/M$ phase by FucciS/G_2/M-#474 mice and G_1 phase by FucciG$_1$-#639 mice without cross-mating is possible.

2. KikGR protein is photoconverted by fluorescent light. KikGR proteins in KikGR mice, particularly in ear are photoconverted during breeding under fluorescent light in the bleeding room. Thus, to avoid photoconversion of KikGR mice, it is required that mouse cages for KikGR mice are shaded from light and located in darker position in cage rack as much as possible. To ensure the reliability of the experiments, it is highly recommended to check breeding condition by confirming no photoconverted cells in ear skin.

3. All of the cells in Kaede mice or KikGR mice express Kaede or KikGR protein. Photoconvertible protein-gene-positive mice could be screened using a handy UV light source. You can observe green fluorescence on the footpad, ear, tail, and other hairless areas of the body by exposing these areas to a handy UV light source. Please make sure that lighting time is minimal. It is recommended to screen in a dark room and compare the Kaede or KikGR mice with wild-type mice. Screening of Kaede or KikGR mice by flow cytometry of peripheral blood lymphocytes is also possible. Fluorescence signals of Kaede or KikGR can be detected using the FITC channel of flow cytometry. Homozygous and heterozygous Kaede or KikGR mice can be distinguished by the difference in the fluorescence intensity.

4. Multicolor flow cytometer is recommended, because FITC and PE channels are used to detect signal from fluorescent proteins.

5. The peak wavelength of photoconverted KikGR protein is 595 nm, thus the filter set for detecting PE is not the best setting. Thus, to detect KikGR-Red signal more efficiently, for example in Fortessa, we changed LP600 and 575/25BP with LP620 and 595/50BP. This filter changes increase signal of KikGR-Red and increase reliability of distinguished non-photoconverted green signal and photoconverted red signal.

6. We chose violet light (435 nm) for photoconversion to minimize damage by light. However, shorter wavelength light (i.e., 405 nm) is more effective for photoconversion of Kaede and KikGR than violet light (436 nm). High power LED (peak wavelength 435 nm or 405 nm) is now available. If you used 405 nm, it is required to check photoconverting condition (strength and time) and damage of the tissue.

7. FITC and PE channels in flow cytometry are used for detection of fluorescence signals of non-photoconverted and photoconverted Kaede or KikGR, respectively. It is difficult to use Tx-Red or PE-Dazzle 594-conjugated antibodies, because signals of photoconverted Kaede and KikGR spill over into Tx-Red channel and compensation for the Tx-Red channel is difficult.

8. In general, excitation wavelength of fluorescent proteins by two-photon laser is broad. Both mKO2 and mAG were excited by two-photon laser at 930 nm. However, excitation efficiencies of mKO2 and mAG are changing along with changing wavelength. You can find the best wavelength that is good balance of mKO2 and mAG signal strength.

9. In general, excitation wavelength of fluorescent proteins by two-photon laser is broad. However, two-photon laser light around 820 nm highly excites ECFP, but not Venus. It makes us possible to detect Venus signal of FRET protein.

10. This way of cutting the skin and visualizing femur minimized interference with the nerve and blood vessels.

11. Cutting both sides and photoconversion of BM from both sides make photoconversion efficiency higher. Bone structure is asymmetric, thus, irradiation from the direction which bone thickness is thin (you can see more red inside the bone from outside) is better to get higher efficiency of photoconversion. However, you should always care about tissue damages.

12. Another instrument is possible.

13. Photoconversion efficiency of cells depends on how much strength of violet light reach to the cell. Using younger mice get better photoconversion efficiency. Because, tissue size is small and bone thickness is thin. Thus violet light is easy to penetrate inside of the bone, where BM cells exist.

14. BM cells and thymocytes are more suitable to set up mAG fluorescent signal. Because, more mAG-positive cells are included in BM cells and thymocytes, while mAG-positive cells are only few in secondary lymphoid organs, such as lymph nodes and spleen [3].

15. In general, small numbers of dead cells are included in culture and samples. You can use these dead cells for control. Sometimes sample includes intermediate cells that are going to die (uncleaved and cleaved SCAT3.1 proteins are included in cell). Signal from SCAT3.1 is disappeared along with loss of plasma membrane integrity because of the release of soluble fluorescent protein SCAT3.1 from cells.

16. Cleavage of SCAT3.1 is enzyme reaction. Thus, when you analyze time course of cell death, samples should be cold (on ice)

immediately at the time point and keep on ice until data acquisition, but analyzing with flow cytometer in real time is the best.

17. For precise gating of non-photoconverted cells and photoconverted cells in analyzing cell subsets, prepare non-photoconverted and photoconverted cells those were stained with appropriate mAbs because (1) signals of non-photoconverted cells in dot plot (x-axis; non-photoconverted, y-axis; photoconverted cells) are different among cell types and (2) a border between photoconverted cells and non-photoconverted cells in measured samples is frequently unobvious.

18. 18 Depended on the mice (particularly size of body) (*see* **Note 13**) and photoconversion condition (*see* **Note 11**), 30–50% of BM cells can be photoconverted (Fig. 1e). A border between photoconverted cells and non-photoconverted cells in BM cells is unobvious, even at immediately after photoconversion. Thus, photoconverted cells are gated by referencing non-photoconverted cells (*see* **Note 17**).

Acknowledgements

This work was supported in part by JSPS Grants-in-Aid for Scientific Research in Innovative Areas "Analysis and Synthesis of Multidimensional Immune Organ Network" (#24111007); JSPS Grants-in-Aid for Scientific Research (B) (#16H05087); Special Coordination Funds for Promoting Science and Technology of the Japanese Government.

References

1. Huang AY, Qi H, Germain RN (2004) Illuminating the landscape of in vivo immunity: insights from dynamic in situ imaging of secondary lymphoid tissues. Immunity 21:331–339

2. Sumen C, Mempel TR, Mazo IB et al (2004) Intravital microscopy: visualizing immunity in context. Immunity 21:315–329

3. Tomura M, Sakaue-Sawano A, Mori Y et al (2013) Contrasting quiescent G_0 phase with mitotic cell cycling in the mouse immune system. PLoS One 8:e73801

4. Tomura M, Mori YS, Watanabe R et al (2009) Time-lapse observation of cellular function with fluorescent probe reveals novel CTL-target cell interactions. Int Immunol 21:1145–1150

5. Tomura M, Yoshida N, Tanaka J et al (2008) Monitoring cellular movement in vivo with photoconvertible fluorescence protein "Kaede" transgenic mice. Proc Natl Acad Sci U S A 105:10871–10876

6. Tomura M, Hata A, Matsuoka S et al (2014) Tracking and quantification of dendritic cell migration and antigen trafficking between the skin and lymph nodes. Sci Rep 4:6030

7. Sakaue-Sawano A, Kurokawa H, Morimura T et al (2008) Visualizing spatiotemporal dynamics of multicellular cell-cycle progression. Cell 132:487–498

8. David R, McIlwain TB, Mak TW (2013) Caspase functions in cell death and disease. Cold Spring Harb Perspect Biol 5:a008656

9. Takemoto K, Nagai T, Miyawaki A et al (2003) Spatio-temporal activation of caspase revealed by indicator that is insensitive to environmental effects. J Cell Biol 160:235–243

10. Nagai T, Miyawaki A (2004) A high-throughput method for development of FRET-based indicators for proteolysis. Biochem Biophys Res Commun 319:72–77

11. Ando R, Hama H, Yamamoto-Hino M et al (2002) An optical marker based on the UV-induced green-to-red photoconversion of a fluorescent protein. Proc Natl Acad Sci U S A 99:12651–12656

12. Tsutsui H, Karasawa S, Shimizu H et al (2005) Semi-rational engineering of a coral fluorescent protein into an efficient highlighter. EMBO Rep 6:233–238

13. Tomura M, Honda T, Tanizaki H et al (2010) Activated regulatory T cells are the major T cell type emigrating from the skin during a cutaneous immune response in mice. J Clin Invest 120:883–893

14. Tomura M, Itoh K, Kanagawa O (2010) Naive CD4+ T lymphocytes circulate through lymphoid organs to interact with endogenous antigens and upregulate their function. J Immunol 184:4646–4653

15. Chtanova T, Hampton HR, Waterhouse LA et al (2014) Real-time interactive two-photon photoconversion of recirculating lymphocytes for discontinuous cell tracking in live adult mice. J Biophotonics 7:425–433. 201

16. Kotani M, Kikuta J, Klauschen F et al (2013) Systemic circulation and bone recruitment of osteoclast precursors tracked by using fluorescent imaging techniques. J Immunol 190:605–612

17. Shand FH, Ueha S, Otsuji M et al (2014) Tracking of intertissue migration reveals the origins of tumor-infiltrating monocytes. Proc Natl Acad Sci U S A 111:7771–7776

18. Ikebuchi R, Teraguchi S, Vandenbon A et al (2016) A rare subset of skin-tropic regulatory T cells expressing *Il10/Gzmb* inhibits the cutaneous immune response. Sci Rep 6:35002

19. Tomura M, Kabashima K (2013) Analysis of cell movement between skin and other anatomical sites in vivo using photoconvertible fluorescent protein "Kaede"-transgenic mice. Mol Dermatol Methods Mol Biol 961:279–286. Spring (Edited by Cristina Has and Cassian Sitaru)

INDEX

Masaru Ishii (ed.), *Intravital Imaging of Dynamic Bone and Immune Systems: Methods and Protocols*, Methods in Molecular Biology, vol. 1763, https://doi.org/10.1007/978-1-4939-7762-8, © Springer Science+Business Media, LLC 2018

Printed in the United States
By Bookmasters